English for the Dental Clinic

音声DL付

歯科医院で使える英語

Jeremy Williams
C.S. Langham　著
井上　孝

医歯薬出版株式会社

本書に付属する音声データについて

・本書中にある 🔊 *1* の番号は，音声データのトラック番号に対応しています．
・本書中に掲載しているQRコードを読み込むと，該当の音声データを再生することができます．
・本書に付属する音声データを下記のURLまたはQRコードから無料でダウンロードすることができます．

https://www.ishiyaku.co.jp/ebooks/456890/

＜注意事項＞
・MP3形式の音声データを再生できる環境が必要です．
・お客様がご負担になる通信料金について十分にご理解のうえご利用をお願いします．
・音声データを無断で複製・公に上映・公衆送信（送信可能化を含む）・翻訳・翻案することは法律により禁止されています．

＜お問合せ先＞
https://www.ishiyaku.co.jp/ebooks/inquiry/

FOREWORD

This book is aimed at dental students and all those working in the dental field interested in using English for dental purposes. The main goal is to introduce some basic dental English that will be of use in communicating with patients.

Each unit contains instructions on how to use the material. However, we know that every student and class is different, and that teachers may come up with new ways of using this material that we hadn't thought of. Therefore, the user should feel free to use this book in any way they like. For example, for a 1st year class in a dental college, this book could be used in conjunction with a standard English textbook. Although there are only 7 units, each unit is quite long. A teacher might use one half of each unit per class, and a teaching schedule might look something like this :

Week 1 : standard English textbook
Week 2 : 1st half of Unit 1 of this book
Week 3 : standard English textbook
Week 4 : 2nd half of Unit 1 of this book
 Etc.

Each unit contains a number of sections in Japanese which can be used to promote general discussion in the case of Japanese-English teachers and a little light relief for the student. We would like to emphasize that this book only contains dental vocabulary intended for the general public. Therefore, there is no need to be a dental specialist to teach this material.

We hope that this textbook will help English teachers combine the teaching of basic English with preparing students for the dental English questions that have now become a part of the national examinations.

Jeremy Williams
C.S. Langham

はじめに

　本書は，歯科医療の現場において，英語を役立てたいと思う歯科医学生達の教育のために書かれたものです．つまり，到達目標は，治療に来る外国人の患者さんと円滑なコミュニケーションをとるために必要な基本的歯科医学英語を修得することです．

　それぞれのユニットでは，どのようにその内容を活用すべきかを述べました．しかし，学生達は十人十色ですし，クラスもそれぞれ状況が違うのは当然のことです．つまり，実際に教えている先生方のほうが，私たちが思いもよらなかった新しい使い方を考えつくかもしれません．結論として，この本をどのように活用するかは使う人次第です．

　例えば，歯科大学の1年目の学生への英語教育であれば，この本と一般的な英会話のテキストを併用することも可能だと思います．全部で7ユニットですが，一つ一つは結構な長さがあります．もし，1回の講義でユニットの半分を使うとすれば，講義内容は次のようにすることも一案です．

第1週：一般的なテキスト
第2週：本書ユニット1の前半
第3週：一般的なテキスト
第4週：本書ユニット1の後半
　etc.

　それぞれのユニットには，ちょっとした日本語の小咄を入れました．そこで内容について少しディスカッションができると，学生たちにも良いコーヒーブレークになるかと思います．

　本書では，患者さんが歯科医院に行って治療してもらう際の，一般的な歯科医学英語のみを収めています．すなわち，歯科の専門家が教えなくてはならないような用語は用いていない事を強調しておきたいと思います．

　最後に，歯科医師国家試験の一部となっている歯科医学英語を教える英語の先生方に，本書が少しでも役立てば幸甚に思います．

著者一同

CONTENTS

1. Your First Set of Teeth ··· ● 2

2. Keeping Your Teeth Looking Nice ························· ● 12

3. Tooth Decay ·· ● 24

4. Dental Implants ··· ● 34

5. Orthodontics ··· ● 44

6. Dental Trauma ·· ● 56

7. Tooth Whitening ·· ● 68

Answer Key ··· ● 79

English for the Dental Clinic

歯科医院で使える英語

Unit1
Your First Set of Teeth

Unit2
Keeping Your Teeth Looking Nice

Unit3
Tooth Decay

Unit4
Dental Implants

Unit5
Orthodontics

Unit6
Dental Trauma

Unit7
Tooth Whitening

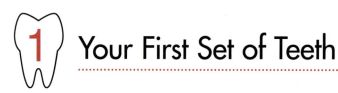

1 Your First Set of Teeth

Part 1 : Vocabulary

Some of these words are just for you : the professional dentist. If you use them to a patient, they may not understand. These words are in red, *italicized* font in the text. Some words you can use among professionals and to patients : these are in ordinary red font.

1) Listen and number the words in the order you hear them 1~13. 🔊 *1*

   primary (　) deciduous (　) permanent (　) baby (　) crown (　)
   erupt (　) shed (　) decay (　) pacifier (　) spit out (　)
   rinse (　) nursing mouth syndrome (　) formula (　)

2)

Step 1 : Repeat these words after you hear them. 🔊 *2*
Step 2 : Study the vocabulary list by yourself for a few minutes.
Step 3 : Make groups of up to 4 students. Test each other : one student chooses an English or Japanese word at random and the other students have to guess the translation.

Note : Don't worry if you do not understand these words, even in translation. Just get used to hearing and saying them.

Vocabulary List

primary　最初の，第一の
deciduous　落葉性の，(ある時期に)抜ける
permanent　永久の
baby　赤ん坊
crown　歯冠
erupt / eruption　萌出する / 萌出
shed / shedding　(自然に) 落ちる，脱落する

decay　う蝕になる / う蝕
pacifier　おしゃぶり
spit out　唾を吐く
rinse　すすぐ
nursing mouth syndrome　哺乳びんう蝕症候群
formula　(乳児用) 人工乳

3) Match the English words with their Japanese translation.

primary ·　　　　　　　　　　　· 歯冠
deciduous ·　　　　　　　　　　· 落葉性の，(ある時期に) 抜ける
permanent ·　　　　　　　　　　· すすぐ
baby ·　　　　　　　　　　　　· 永久の
crown ·　　　　　　　　　　　　· 萌出する / 萌出
erupt / eruption ·　　　　　　　· 赤ん坊
shed / shedding ·　　　　　　　· (自然に) 落ちる，脱落する
decay ·　　　　　　　　　　　　· 唾を吐く
pacifier ·　　　　　　　　　　　· (乳児用) 人工乳
spit out ·　　　　　　　　　　　· う蝕になる / う蝕
rinse ·　　　　　　　　　　　　· おしゃぶり
nursing mouth syndrome ·　　　　· 哺乳びんう蝕症候群
formula ·　　　　　　　　　　　· 最初の，第一の

4) Listen and write down the words you hear. 🔊 *3*

1. _____　2. _____
3. _____　4. _____.
5. _____.

Part 2 : Reading

Note : Reading strategy

Step 1 : Just read through as quickly as you can. Do not use your dictionary.

Step 2 : Read again more slowly. Underline any words you do not know. Use your dictionary *after* you have finished reading. Do not try to memorize more than a few words at one go.

Step 3 : Read through again at normal speed.

Your First Set of Teeth

Most people do not realize that they are actually born with teeth! Your first set of teeth are called the "*primary*" or "*deciduous*" teeth, and will eventually be replaced by "*permanent*" teeth. The dentist usually calls the primary teeth "baby" teeth when talking to a mother. By the time you are born, the crowns of all 20 of these baby teeth are fully formed. However, they are hidden in the infant's jawbones. They will begin to erupt at around 6 months. First to appear will be the two upper and two lower front teeth. They should all have erupted by the age of 3 years.

From the age of around 6 years onwards, you will start to shed the primary teeth and the permanent teeth will begin to appear. This will take a few years, usually until around the age of 12 years, as the jaw needs time to grow large enough to contain all 32 of them. Each tooth has a name depending on its position and function (see diagram).

The primary teeth are very important. Of course, the child will need them to eat with, but they have two other important functions too : first, they are necessary for language ; second, they keep a place ready for the permanent tooth that will replace them. All this means that they should be looked after with great care.

Some mothers do not realize that they need to look after their baby's teeth. They think they are only temporary, so not important. But this is not true : tooth decay in the primary teeth can affect the permanent teeth which are growing just beneath them.

There are two things, in particular, that the mother can do to help prevent tooth

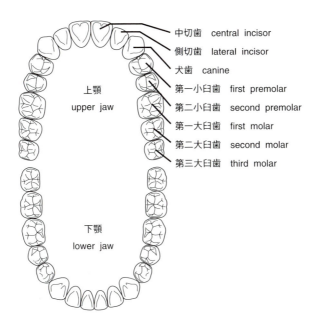

decay : first, she can make sure that the baby doesn't fall asleep with the feeding bottle still in its mouth ; second, she can make sure not to dip the baby's pacifier in something sweet such as honey or sugar.

After feeding, the mother should wipe the baby's gums with a wet cloth. When teeth begin to appear, she can also brush them with a little water. As the child gets older and the number of teeth increases, she can make sure that he or she learns how to clean them properly, making sure to spit out the toothpaste after and rinse thoroughly with water.

If she does all of this, then the baby should avoid what we call "baby bottle" tooth decay or "nursing mouth syndrome", which occurs due to long exposure to sugary liquids such as milk, formula or fruit juice.

Read 1

Fast Facts : Read through the passage quickly and complete this grid. Then check your answers with a partner.

1. Your first teeth are called _____ or _____ teeth by a dentist. 2. Your second teeth are called _____ teeth. 3. Dentists use the word _____ teeth when talking with a mother about the first set of teeth. 4. Primary teeth first appear by the age of _____. 5. All primary teeth should have erupted by the age of_____. 6. Children will start shedding teeth at the age of _____. 7. Children will finish shedding teeth by the age of _____. 8. Primary teeth are needed for _____ and _____ and to keep a _____ ready for the permanent tooth. 9. Tooth decay in primary teeth can _____ the permanent teeth. 10. Nursing mouth syndrome occurs when babies are exposed to _____ _____ for long periods.

Read 2

How much did you understand?

Answer true (T) or false (F) to each of these statements :
1. Your permanent teeth will soon be replaced by deciduous teeth. ( )
2. The crowns of all your baby teeth are fully formed by the age of 6 years. ( )
3. The primary teeth will erupt at around 6 months. ( )
4. The deciduous teeth should be well looked after. ( )
5. Tooth decay in the primary teeth can not affect the permanent teeth. ( )
6. The mother should wipe the baby's gums after feeding. ( )
7. Nursing mouth syndrome occurs after long exposure to toothpaste. ( )

Read 3

Let's answer : Now try and answer these questions based on the text.

1. Why does it take until 12 years of age for all the permanent teeth to erupt?
2. You need the primary teeth to eat with. What else do you need them for?
3. Why do some mothers think that the baby teeth are not important?
4. What should the mother make sure the baby does not do?
5. What should she do after feeding?

Listening

Number focus : Listen to the text and circle the correct number in each of the sentences 1~5. 🔊 *4*

1. By the time they are born, babies will have (20 / 32) primary teeth.
2. Primary teeth should all have erupted by the age of (6 months / 3 years / 6 years).
3. Children start to shed their primary teeth at the age of (3 / 6 / 12) years.
4. Children will finish shedding their teeth at the age of (3 / 6 / 12) years.
5. Later the child will have (20 / 32) permanent teeth.

 Coffee Break

　人間では 20 本の乳歯が生え揃うのは 3 歳前後である．その後，永久歯に生え換わり，28 ～ 32 本の永久歯列になる．28 ～ 32 本と幅があるのは，近代人間では，親知らずが退化する傾向にあるからである．一方，サメの歯は抜けても何度でも生え換わる．われわれ哺乳類は一度だけ乳歯から永久歯に生え換わるが，その後歯を失えば入れ歯やインプラントに頼らざるをえない．2011 年，マウスでは幹細胞から歯をつくる再生歯ができるようになったが，ヒトではまだ 10 年は待たないとできそうにないと報告があった．

Part 3 : Dialogue

1) Preliminary listening exercises

Keywords : Here are 12 keywords from the dialogue. Listen and number them in the order you hear them. 🔊 *5*

erupt (　) fall out (　) tooth decay (　) avoid (　) wipe (　) gums (　) wet cloth (　) feeding (　) brush (　) meals (　) spit out (　) rinse (　)

Question focus : The mother asks the dentist 5 questions. Listen and complete the questions. 🔊 *6*

1. _____ _____ will it take for the others to appear?
2. _____ _____ that a problem?
3. _____ _____ I avoid that?
4. _____ _____ clean the teeth that have erupted?
5. _____ _____ I do when he is a little older and has more teeth?

2) Listening

Cover the dialogue below and just listen two or three times. Finally, number these sentences in the order that you hear them 1~5. 🔊 *7*

1. You should always wipe his gums with a wet cloth after feeding. (　)
2. You should teach him to brush after meals. (　)
3. Yes, but decay in the baby teeth can affect the permanent teeth. (　)
4. Yes, but not just milk : things like formula and fruit juice. This can cause tooth decay. (　)
5. How long will it take for the others to appear? (　)

3) **Activity**

Step 1 : Read the dialogue below. Use your dictionary and ask your teacher if there is anything you do not understand. When you have read and understood the dialogue, take turns reading each part with a partner. Try this : 1) Look at each line. 2) Cover each line. 3) Read each line without looking.

In the clinic : Educating mother

Parent : Tom's first tooth has appeared. I wanted to see if it was OK.

Dentist : Well, let's take a look. Yes, this appears to be fine.

Parent : How long will it take for the others to appear?

Dentist : The rest of the baby teeth should erupt over the next 2 years or so.

Parent : Well, no problem. I guess they will all fall out anyway.

Dentist : Well, they will all fall out, but you should still be very careful with them.

Parent : Why?

Dentist : Well, babies often drink a lot of sugary liquids.

Parent : You mean milk?

Dentist : Yes, but not just milk : things like formula and fruit juice. This can cause tooth decay.

Parent : Why is that a problem? He will get permanent teeth later anyway.

Dentist : Yes, but decay in the baby teeth can affect the permanent teeth.

Parent : How should I avoid that? He has to eat *something*.

Dentist : Well, there are several things you can do. You should always wipe his gums with a wet cloth after feeding.

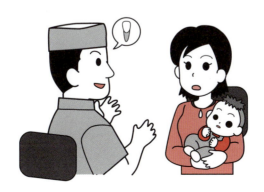

Parent : OK. Should I clean the teeth that have erupted?
Dentist : Yes, but only with a little water.
Parent : What should I do when he is a little older and has more teeth?
Dentist : You should teach him to brush after meals.
Parent : Anything else?
Dentist : Yes, make sure he spits out the toothpaste and rinses thoroughly with water after brushing.

Step 2 : Now take turns playing the dentist or the patient. Your questions and answers do not have to be exactly the same as in the dialogue above.

Tip : Did you notice we used the patterns "You should" and "Make sure you / he does" a lot? Try to use these patterns in answering the mother.

Word stew

Can you unscramble these words?

marirpy
ciduodeus
rconw
turep
yedca

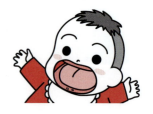

Micro-presentation

In a group list up the things mothers should and should not do in order to keep their babies' teeth healthy. Then practice a short presentation.

Tales from the clinic

　歯の萌出には順番がある．乳歯では，下顎の乳中切歯が生後6，7カ月で，次いで上顎の乳中切歯が生後8〜11カ月で生えてくる．その次は下顎の乳側切歯が10〜12カ月で，そして上顎の乳側切歯が11〜12カ月で，その後は上下ほぼ同じ時期に，1歳8カ月くらいで乳犬歯と第一乳臼歯が，2歳で第二乳臼歯が生えてくる．永久歯への生え換わりでは，中切歯は乳中切歯の位置に生え，側切歯は乳側切歯の位置に，犬歯は乳犬歯の位置に生えてくる．第一小臼歯は第一乳臼歯の位置に，第二小臼歯は第二乳臼歯の位置に生えてくる．第一大臼歯の部位に乳歯はなく，乳歯の奥に生え，第二大臼歯は第一大臼歯の後方に生える．

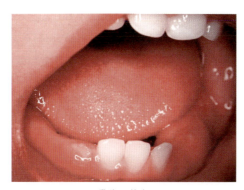

乳歯の萌出

2 Keeping Your Teeth Looking Nice

Part 1 : Vocabulary

Some of these words are just for you : the professional dentist. If you use them to a patient, they may not understand. These words are in red, *italicized* font in the text. Some words you can use among professionals and to patients : these are in ordinary red font.

1) Listen and number the words in the order you hear them 1~12. 🔊 *8*

   saliva ( ) inflammation ( ) tartar ( ) calculus ( ) plaque ( ) bulimia ( ) floss ( ) colonize ( ) soft-bristled ( ) calcify ( ) stroke ( ) species ( )

2)

Step 1 : Repeat these words after you hear them. 🔊 *9*

Step 2 : Study the vocabulary list by yourself for a few minutes.

Step 3 : Make groups of up to 4 students. Test each other : one student chooses an English or Japanese word at random and the other students have to guess the translation.

Note : Don't worry if you do not understand these words, even in translation. Just get used to hearing and saying them.

Vocabulary List

floss　デンタルフロスを使う，絹糸	soft-bristled　柔らかい毛の
plaque　プラーク	stroke　ストローク，(一連の動作の) 一動き
saliva　唾液	inflammation　炎症
colonize　コロニー（集落）をつくる	bulimia　過食症，食欲異常亢進
species　種族	binge eating　過食，大食
calcify　石灰化する	anorexia nervosa　神経性食欲不振，拒食症
calculus　歯石，結石	systemic　全身的な
tartar　歯石，酒石	

3) Match the English words with their Japanese translation.

floss ·	· 全身的な
plaque ·	· プラーク
saliva ·	· デンタルフロスを使う，絹糸
colonize ·	· 唾液
species ·	· ストローク，(一連の動作の) 一動き
calcify ·	· 柔らかい毛の
calculus ·	· 歯石，結石
tartar ·	· コロニー（集落）をつくる
soft-bristled ·	· 種族
stroke ·	· 神経性食欲不振，拒食症
inflammation ·	· 炎症
bulimia ·	· 石灰化する
binge eating ·	· 歯石，酒石
anorexia nervosa ·	· 過食，大食
systemic ·	· 過食症，食欲異常亢進

4) Listen and write down the words you hear. 🔊 *10*

1. _____.　2. _____.
3. _____.　4. _____.
5. _____.

Part 2 : Reading

Note : Reading strategy

Step 1 : Just read through as quickly as you can. Do not use your dictionary.

Step 2 : Read again more slowly. Underline any words you do not know. Use your dictionary *after* you have finished reading. Do not try to memorize more than a few words at one go.

Step 3 : Read through again at normal speed.

Keeping Your Teeth Looking Nice

Keeping your teeth looking nice is important. To do this, there are just three things you need to remember : brushing, flossing and diet. If you are careful about all three, your teeth should be safe from plaque, the number one enemy of oral health.

Plaque starts to form within minutes on a tooth that has just been cleaned. First, elements of saliva form a sticky layer on the tooth, which is then colonized by many species of bacteria. It is soft and yellowish in appearance, at first, and can be removed with a toothbrush. Later, though, it will calcify, meaning harden, and form *calculus*, or tartar. Now it can only be removed by a dentist. The problem is that bacteria in the plaque will use sugars in your diet to produce acid, which then causes tooth decay.

Your main weapon against plaque is brushing. You should brush your teeth twice a day after meals. It is best to use a soft-bristled toothbrush and fluoride toothpaste. You should also learn proper brushing technique.

You should keep the toothbrush at a 45-degree angle to the gums and move it back and forth in short strokes. Do not brush too hard, as this may irritate the gums and cause inflammation. Brush gently. Make sure you brush the chewing surfaces of the teeth, as well as the inner and outer surfaces. Reaching the inner surfaces can be difficult. Use the tip of the toothbrush to reach them and move the brush in an up-down stroke. You should also gently brush your tongue, as this will help remove bacteria and keep your breath smelling fresh.

You have many choices for flossing. For example, you can use a line of floss or

14 ● Unit 2 Keeping Your Teeth Looking Nice

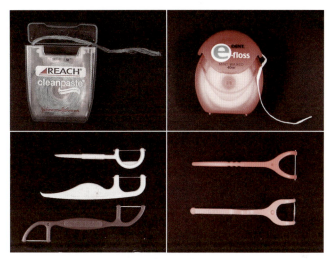

フロスにはさまざまな形状のものがある

you can buy floss already attached to a bow (See picture). Whichever you choose, move the floss gently between your teeth toward your gums. Never let it snap into your gums, as this could damage them. When it reaches the gums, bend it into a C-shape and start to pull it back and forth while moving away from the gum toward the tip of the tooth. Then repeat between the next pair of teeth. You should do this once a day. As an alternative, you can also use an interdental brush.

Finally, you should be careful about your diet. Snacking and consumption of sweet drinks will increase the amount of acid on your teeth. Eating disorders such as bulimia, binge eating and anorexia nervosa can also have a bad effect on both systemic and oral health. So eat a balanced diet.

Remember, though : acid may be damaging your teeth without you knowing it. So see your dentist often if you want to keep that beautiful smile.

Read 1

Fast Facts : Read through the passage quickly and complete this grid. Then check your answers with a partner.

1. To keep your teeth looking nice, you must remember _____, _____ and diet. 2. This is because _____ is the biggest enemy of oral health. 3. Plaque begins to form within _____ of brushing your teeth. 4. First, elements of _____ form a _____ _____ on the tooth. This is then _____ by bacteria. Later, it will _____ and form _____ or _____. 5. Your main weapon against plaque is _____. 6. Do not brush too hard, as it might _____ the gums. 7. As an alternative, you can _____ your teeth or use an _____ brush. 8. You should also be careful about your _____. 9. Avoid _____ between meals. 10. Eating disorders such as _____ can also affect your oral health.

Read 2

How much did you understand?

Answer true (T) or false (F) to each of these statements :

1. The three most important things to remember are brushing, flossing and diet. ( )
2. Plaque starts to form within hours of cleaning your teeth. ( )
3. Calculus can be removed by brushing. ( )
4. It is best to use a soft-bristled brush. ( )
5. Plaque is formed by elements of saliva sticking to your tooth. ( )
6. Later this layer will calcify and form a soft yellowish layer on the tooth. ( )
7. Bacteria in the plaque will use sugars in your diet to produce acid. ( )

Read 3

Let's answer : Now try and answer these questions based on the text.

1. What angle should you keep your toothbrush at?
2. Why should you be careful to not brush too hard?
3. Which three surfaces of the tooth should you brush?
4. Which part of the brush should you use to reach the inner surfaces?
5. What else should you brush?
6. When you insert floss between your teeth, which direction should you move it at first?
7. What should you never let it do?
8. When you start to pull it back and forth, which direction should you move in?

Listening

Word focus : Listen to this extract from the text a few times and circle the correct word in each of the sentences 1 ~ 6. 🔊 *11*

1. You should keep the toothbrush at a (four or five / forty-five) degree angle.
2. (Reaching / bleaching) the inner surfaces can be difficult.
3. Move the brush in an (uptown / up-down) stroke.
4. You should also gently brush your tongue, as this will help you (move / remove) bacteria.
5. Then (repeat / read eat) between the next pair of teeth.
6. As an alternative, you can also use an (incidental / interdental) brush.

Part 3 : Dialogue

1) Preliminary listening exercises

Keywords : Here are 9 keywords from the dialogue. Listen and number them in the order you hear them. 🔊 *12*

buildup ( ) fluoride ( ) bow-type ( ) smelling ( ) hard-bristled ( ) angle ( ) irritate ( ) pairs ( ) plaque ( )

Question focus : The dentist gives the patient some information and advice. Listen and complete what the dentist says. 🔊 *13*

1. You need to brush them _____ _____.
2. _____ _____ use a soft-bristled brush.
3. You should _____ the toothbrush at a 45-degree angle toward the gum.
4. You should move it _____ and _____ in short strokes, like this.
5. _____ _____ too hard, as that might irritate the gums.
6. _____ _____ the bow-type floss, as it is easier to use.
7. _____ the floss between your teeth and move it gently toward your gum.
8. Then move the floss _____ and _____ while moving toward the tip of the tooth.

2) Listening

Cover the dialogue below and just listen two or three times. Finally, number these sentences in the order that you hear them 1~6. 🔊 *14*

1. I have never flossed before. How do you do it? ( )
2. Should I move it up and down? ( )
3. What kind of a toothbrush do you use? ( )
4. OK. Anything else? ( )
5. How should I brush the inner surfaces of the teeth? ( )
6. I use my local supermarket brand. ( )

3) **Activity**

Step 1 : Read the dialogue below. Use your dictionary and ask your teacher if there is anything you do not understand. When you have read and understood the dialogue, take turns reading each part with a partner. Try this : 1) Look at each line. 2) Cover each line. 3) Read each line without looking.

In the clinic : Keeping Your Teeth Looking Nice

Dentist : Well, you are starting to get a buildup of plaque on your teeth. You need to brush them more carefully.

Patient : How?

Dentist : What kind of a toothbrush do you use?

Patient : I use a hard-bristled brush.

Dentist : You should use a soft-bristled brush. What kind of toothpaste do you use?

Patient : I use my local supermarket brand.

Dentist : Well, it is best to use fluoride toothpaste. Now, please show me how you brush your teeth.

Patient : OK.

Dentist : Mm. That's not so good. You should hold the toothbrush at a 45-degree angle toward the gum, like this.

Patient : Should I move it up and down?

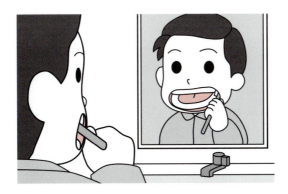

Dentist : No, you should move it back and forth in short strokes, like this.

Patient : How should I brush the inner surfaces of the teeth? I find that difficult.

Dentist : You should use the tip of the toothbrush, like this. You should move the toothbrush up and down, like this.

Patient : Is there anything else?

Dentist : Don't brush too hard, as that might irritate the gums. You should brush gently.

Patient : OK.

Dentist : Oh, and you can also brush your tongue.

Patient : Why?

Dentist : That will help get rid of bacteria and keep your breath smelling fresh. You should also floss. I recommend the bow-type floss, as it is easier to use.

Patient : I have never flossed before. How do you do it?

Dentist : Slide the floss between your teeth and move it gently toward your gum. Then move the floss back and forth while moving toward the tip of the tooth. Repeat between all pairs of teeth.

Patient : OK. Anything else?

Dentist : Yes, try to avoid snacking and soft drinks as they provide food for bacteria. And don't forget to see me regularly for a checkup!

Grammar note :

There are many patterns for giving advice and instructions in English. If you are giving instructions on a process, like using a public phone, for example, you can just use the verb :

Pick up the phone. Dial the number. Insert the money.

You don't need to use phrases like "You should" or "You have to". However, if you want to be a little more polite, you can use "You should". There are many more ways to give advice, but they are more difficult to use properly :

You should brush your teeth gently. You shouldn't brush too hard. You should use fluoride toothpaste. You shouldn't snack.

Another way to give advice on what not to do is to use the pattern "You should avoid doing X" :

You should avoid snacking. You should avoid soft drinks.

Step 2 : Now take turns playing the dentist or the patient. Your questions and answers do not have to be exactly the same as in the dialogue above.

Word stew

Can you unscramble these words?

puilbud
eglna
ozocleni
llcsacuu
sciepes

21

Micro-presentation

In a group, make a list of the main things to remember about brushing and flossing. Then practice giving a short presentation on this topic.

Tales from the clinic

　歯石は，歯に付着したプラークが石灰化したもので，容易に除去できない歯の沈着物である．歯肉縁より上にできるものを歯肉縁上歯石，歯肉縁より下にできるものを歯肉縁下歯石といい，それぞれ性質が異なる．歯石自体には病原性はないとされるが，新たなプラークが付着しやすくなるため，歯周疾患の原因とされ，歯石の除去は歯周治療においてとても重要である．

　歯磨きは，歯や歯茎に対してブラッシングを行い，歯垢などの汚れを落とす作業のことをいう．実際は歯を磨いているわけではなく，歯科領域ではブラッシングとよぶことを推奨している．歯磨きに使う練り歯磨き剤などを「歯磨き粉」とよぶ．チューブタイプの練り歯磨き以前の製品はパウダー状であり「粉」という呼称はその頃の名残である．また，歯磨剤自体のことを「ハミガキ」とよぶこともある．

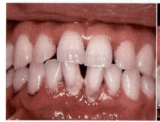 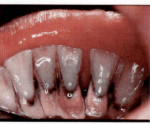 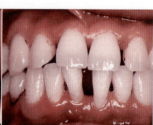

歯石がついた歯列（唇側面）　　歯石がついた歯列（舌側面）　　歯石除去後の歯列

Coffee Break

　歯のみならず，口腔内をきれいに保つことは，全身の健康にもおおいに役に立つ．健康とは，よく食べられ，よく眠れ，風邪をひかず，あまり疲れないことをいう（WHO）．口の中が汚いと，歯と歯肉の間から細菌が体のなかに侵入し，これが動脈硬化や糖尿病などの病気と関係が深いことが明らかとなった．最近では，歯肉の炎症により産生されるCRPというタンパク質が肥満と関係があるともいわれている．

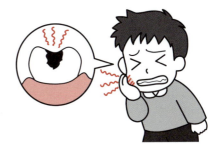

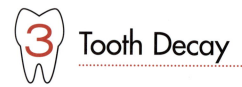

3 Tooth Decay

Part 1 : Vocabulary

Some of these words are just for you : the professional dentist. If you use them to a patient, they may not understand. These words are in red, *italicized* font in the text. Some words you can use among professionals and to patients : these are in ordinary red font.

1) Listen and number the words in the order you hear them 1~13. 🔊 *15*

enamel ( ) debris ( ) porous ( ) virulence factors ( ) caries ( )
accumulate ( ) filling ( ) dentin ( ) carbohydrates ( ) consult ( )
nerve ( ) dental hygiene ( ) tooth decay ( )

2)

Step 1 : Repeat these words after you hear them. 🔊 *16*
Step 2 : Study the vocabulary list by yourself for a few minutes.
Step 3 : Make groups of up to 4 students. Test each other : one student chooses an English or Japanese word at random and the other students have to guess the translation.

Note : Don't worry if you do not understand these words, even in translation. Just get used to hearing and saying them.

Vocabulary List

tooth decay　う蝕	lifestyle　生活様式
filling　充填材，詰め物	snack　軽食をとる，軽食，間食
be treated　処置される	dental hygiene　歯科衛生
caries　う蝕	debris　食物残渣
be vulnerable to something　何かに対して弱い，何かに攻撃されやすい	accumulate　蓄積する
	enamel　エナメル質
bacterium / bacteria　細菌	calcium　カルシウム
Mutans streptococcus　ストレプトコッカス スミュータンス	dentin　象牙質
	nerve　神経
virulence factors　病原性因子	tissue　組織
adhere to something　何かに付着する	pulp　歯髄
acid　酸	consult your dentist　歯科医に診察してもらう
rot　腐敗 / 腐敗する	
diet　食生活	porous　穴のあいた，多孔性の
carbohydrates　炭水化物	

3) Match the English words with their Japanese translation.

rot ·	· 軽食をとる，軽食，間食
carbohydrates ·	· 組織
lifestyle ·	· 生活様式
snack ·	· カルシウム
debris ·	· 食物残渣
enamel ·	· エナメル質
nerve ·	· 腐敗 / 腐敗する
calcium ·	· 神経
tissue ·	· 歯髄
pulp ·	· 炭水化物

4) Listen and write down the word you hear. 🔊 *17*

1. _____．　2. _____．
3. _____．　4. _____．
5. _____．

● 25

Part 2 : Reading

Note : Reading strategy :

Step 1 : Just read through as quickly as you can. Do not use your dictionary.

Step 2 : Read again more slowly. Underline any words you do not know. Use your dictionary *after* you have finished reading. Do not try to memorize more than a few words at one go.

Step 3 : Read through again at normal speed.

Tooth Decay

Fifty years ago, tooth decay was a big problem, especially in children, and almost everybody had to have a filling by the time they reached adulthood. Thanks to our understanding of how tooth decay occurs, this has changed, but people still get tooth decay and need to be treated.

The dentist calls this condition *caries*. So what causes caries and why are children vulnerable to caries, in particular? Well, caries is caused by bacteria, and especially the bacterium *Mutans streptococcus*. This particular bacterium has three weapons, or what we call *virulence factors*, to attack our teeth with. First, it can adhere to our teeth very strongly, so it doesn't get washed away when we drink or rinse our mouths. Second, it can produce much higher amounts of acid from sugar than other bacteria. Third, it is tough : the acid it produces doesn't kill it.

Now, you will often hear people say things like, "Oh, eating sweets will rot your teeth." But this is only partly true : it is not the sugar that rots your teeth ; it is the acid produced by bacteria, which live on that sugar. To make matters worse, the modern diet is rich in carbohydrates, which is the ideal food for such bacteria.

Another problem is our modern lifestyle. Many people go all day without cleaning their teeth. Worse still, they often snack between meals. This poor dental hygiene means that food debris has time to accumulate between your teeth, making a kind of supermarket for the bacteria!

So what about children? Well, people often say things like, "Oh, bacteria will eat their way through your tooth." Again, this is not quite true. Bacteria actually

26 ● Unit 3 Tooth Decay

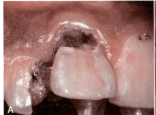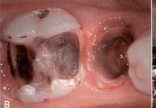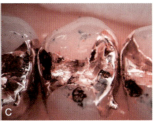

　う蝕（虫歯）とは，口腔内の細菌が糖質から作った酸によって，歯質を脱灰して起こる歯の実質欠損のことである（Aの切歯，Bの大臼歯）．歯周病と並び，歯科の二大疾患の１つである．う蝕は風邪と同様，どの世代でも抱える一般的な病気である．特に歯の萌出後の数年は石灰化度が低いためう蝕になりやすく，未成年に多くみられる．う蝕は硬組織の欠損であり，金属（C）やプラスチックで修復する．

destroy the tooth from the inside. This is because the enamel of a deciduous tooth has many tiny cracks, and is much thinner than the enamel of a permanent tooth. Therefore, the bacteria are able to get inside the tooth, where they produce acid, which eats away the supporting calcium of the enamel and the *dentin* underneath that.

　The problem here is that there is no pain at first, because the nerves of the tooth are in the innermost *tissue*, the *pulp*. Therefore, by the time you notice pain, the damage has already been done. This is why you should always consult your dentist regularly, even if you don't have toothache.

　In older people, the enamel is less porous and thicker, making it much more difficult for this to occur, although not impossible.

 Coffee Break

　歯にできるう蝕（虫歯）は皮膚にできる傷と同じように考えられる．人体の表面はすべて上皮により覆われており，歯とて例外ではない．しかし，歯の場合には機能的な面から上皮が硬質化しエナメル質となり，物をかみ砕くことができるようになった．さて，上皮に欠損が起こるような傷ができると，そこからは，上皮下の血管結合組織が露出し，細菌が入り，感染の侵入門戸となる．歯のエナメル質もう蝕により脱灰されると，エナメル質はなくなり，その下の象牙質が現れる．象牙質は血管結合組織の仲間であるから，そこは炎症の場となる．つまり歯がしみたり，痛くなったりするのである．

Read 1

Fast Facts : Read through the passage quickly and complete this grid. Then check your answers with a partner.

1. Fifty years ago almost everybody had to have a _____ because of _____ _____. 2. The dentist calls this _____. 3. It is caused by _____, especially _____ _____. 4. This particular bacterium has what we call _____ _____. 5. It can _____ to your teeth. 6. It produces more _____ than other bacteria, and it can live in that environment. 7. The modern diet is full of _____. 8. The bacteria in your mouth produce _____, which destroys your teeth. 9. There is no pain at first, because the nerves are in the innermost _____, the _____. 10. Therefore, you should _____ your dentist often. 11. Older people are less vulnerable to caries because the enamel of their teeth is less _____.

Read 2

How much did you understand?

Answer true (T) or false (F) to each of these statements :

1. People still get tooth decay, but don't need to be treated. ( )
2. Children are vulnerable to caries, in particular. ( )
3. The modern diet has too many carbohydrates. ( )
4. Poor dental hygiene means debris doesn't accumulate in your mouth. ( )
5. The innermost layer of your tooth is the dentin. ( )
6. There are no nerves in enamel. ( )
7. The enamel in children is less porous than that in adults. ( )

28 ● Unit 3 Tooth Decay

Read 3

Let's answer : Now try and answer these questions based on the text.

1. Why did most people need a filling fifty years ago?
2. What are the three virulence factors of *Mutans streptococcus*?
3. What is the problem with our modern lifestyle?
4. How do bacteria get inside the tooth?
5. Why is there no pain at first?

Listening

Word focus : Listen to this extract from the text a few times and circle the correct word in each of the sentences 1~5. 🔊 *18*

1. The dentist calls this condition (cherries / caries).
2. This particular bacterium has 3 weapons, or what we call (virulence / violence) factors.
3. It can (add hair / adhere) to our teeth very strongly.
4. Second, it can produce much (higher / tighter) amounts of acid from sugar.
5. To make matters worse, the modern diet is (reaching / rich in) carbohydrates.

Part 3 : Dialogue

1) Preliminary listening exercises

Keywords : Here are 11 keywords from the dialogue. Listen and number them in the order you hear them. 🔊 *19*

interdental ( ) pulp ( ) checkup ( ) bacteria ( ) tooth decay ( ) hygiene ( ) pain ( ) snacking ( ) diet ( ) floss ( ) fluoride ( )

Question focus : The dentist gives the patient's mother some information and advice. Listen and complete what the dentist says. 🔊 *20*

1. You should _____ young Tom _____ for regular checkups.
2. Yes, but he could be _____ tooth decay.
3. There would be no pain until the bacteria _____ the _____.
4. Snacking is a big _____ of _____ _____.
5. Use _____ toothpaste.
6. Also, make him _____ his teeth or use an _____ brush.
7. Just remember : _____, _____, regular checkups.

2) Listening

Cover the dialogue below and just listen two or three times. Finally, number these sentences in the order you hear them 1~5. 🔊 *21*

1. But don't let him eat between meals. ( )
2. His teeth look fine, and he has no pain. ( )
3. Should I let him eat sweets and ice cream? ( )
4. Is there anything else you suggest? ( )
5. Because bacteria can get inside the tooth and destroy it from the inside out. ( )

3) **Activity**

Step 1 : Read the dialogue below. Use your dictionary and ask your teacher if there is anything you do not understand. When you have read and understood the dialogue, take turns reading each part with a partner. Try this : 1) Look at each line. 2) Cover each line. 3) Read each line without looking.

In the clinic : Tooth decay

Dentist : You know, you should bring young Tom in for regular checkups.
Patient's mother : But why? His teeth look fine, and he has no pain.
Dentist : Yes, but he could be getting tooth decay. You just can't see it yet.
Patient's mother : Why not?
Dentist : Because bacteria can get inside the tooth and destroy it from the inside out.
Patient's mother : But wouldn't that be painful?
Dentist : No, not at first. There would be no pain until the bacteria reached the pulp. And then it is too late.
Patient's mother : Oh, no! Is he OK?
Dentist : Hc's OK for now, but you must take care.
Patient's mother : Is there anything I can do to prevent him from getting tooth decay?
Dentist : Yes. First, control his diet.
Patient's mother : Should I let him eat sweets and ice cream?
Dentist : Yes, that is OK. But don't let him eat between meals. Snacking is a big cause of tooth decay.

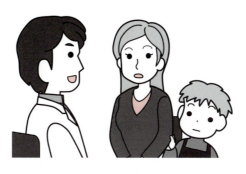

Patient's mother : Why? How is that different to eating sweets at mealtimes?

Dentist : It's a problem of dental hygiene. Of course, you can make him clean his teeth after meals. But you probably can't make him clean his teeth after a snack. This provides food for the bacteria that cause tooth decay.

Patient's mother : Is there anything else you suggest?

Dentist : Yes. Use fluoride toothpaste. Also, make him floss his teeth or use an interdental brush.

Patient's mother : Will he be OK if I do all that?

Dentist : Probably, yes. Just remember : diet, hygiene, regular checkups.

Vocabulary Notes

- fluoride　フッ化物, フッ素化合物
- floss　フロス, デンタルフロス
- interdental brush　歯間ブラシ

Step 2 : Now take turns playing the dentist or the patient. Your questions and answers do not have to be exactly the same as in the dialogue above.

Word stew

Can you unscramble these words?

sbderi
iserac
uceenirvl
tor
ssueit

Micro-presentation

In a group, make a note of why you should consult your dentist regularly to avoid tooth decay in children. Then practice giving a short presentation.

Tales from the clinic

　う蝕は，小窩裂溝う蝕（小窩裂溝部は清掃を行いにくく，食物残渣がたまりやすいため，う蝕が多く見られる；A），平滑面う蝕（歯頸部や隣接面にみられるう蝕．隣接面う蝕はエックス線撮影で明らかになることが多い；B），そして，根面う蝕（歯肉が退縮し，食物残渣がたまりやすい部分が露出することにより発生．高齢者に多い；C）に分類される．治療をせず放置すれば，やがて歯髄に炎症がおよび，最悪の場合には歯を失うことにもなりかねない．

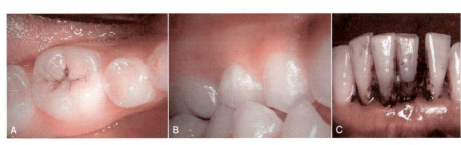

小窩裂溝う蝕　　　　　　　平滑面う蝕　　　　　　　根面う蝕

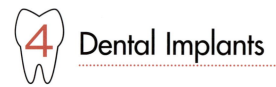

4 Dental Implants

Part 1 : Vocabulary

Some of these words are just for you : the professional dentist. If you use them to a patient, they may not understand. These words are in red, *italicized* font in the text. Some words you can use among professionals *and* to patients : these are in ordinary red font.

1) Listen and number the words in the order you hear them 1~13. 🔊 *22*

alloy ( ) esthetic ( ) titanium ( ) mandible ( ) trauma ( )
crown ( ) osseointegration ( ) maxilla ( ) removable dentures ( )
anchor ( ) temporomandibular joint ( ) dental implant ( )
partial dentures ( )

2)

Step 1 : Repeat these words after you hear them. 🔊 *23*
Step 2 : Study the vocabulary list by yourself for a few minutes.
Step 3 : Make groups of up to 4 students. Test each other : one student chooses an English or Japanese word at random and the other students have to guess the translation.

Note : Don't worry if you do not understand these words, even in translation. Just get used to hearing and saying them.

Vocabulary List

disease 病気	tooth root 歯根
trauma 外傷	mandible 下顎
esthetic 審美的な	maxilla 上顎
crown クラウン	anchor something to something 何かを何かに固定する
removable denture 可撤性義歯	
dental implant 歯科インプラント	osseointegration オッセオインテグレーション
titanium チタン，チタニウム	
alloy 合金	oral hygiene 口腔衛生
fuse to something 何かと結合する	drawback 不利な点，欠点
partial or full denture 部分床義歯または全部床義歯	temporomandibular joint 顎関節
	chew 咬む

3) Match the English words with their Japanese translation.

esthetic ·   · 合金
crown ·   · 上顎
temporomandibular joint ·   · 下顎
partial denture ·   · 可撤性義歯
alloy ·   · 不利な点，欠点
osseointegration ·   · オッセオインテグレーション
oral hygiene ·   · 口腔衛生
chew ·   · 審美的な
drawback ·   · 顎関節
mandible ·   · 咬む
tooth root ·   · 歯根
maxilla ·   · クラウン
removable denture ·   · 部分床義歯

4) Listen and write down the words you hear. 🔊 *24*

1. _____.   2. _____.
3. _____.   4. _____.
5. _____.

● 35

Part 2 : Reading

Note : Reading strategy

Step 1 : Just read through as quickly as you can. Do not use your dictionary.

Step 2 : Read again more slowly. Underline any words you do not know. Use your dictionary *after* you have finished reading. Do not try to memorize more than a few words at one go.

Step 3 : Read through again at normal speed.

Dental Implants

One day you may lose a tooth or some teeth due to disease or trauma. This can cause esthetic problems, meaning it doesn't look nice. More seriously, it may even affect your ability to speak or eat.

For many years, the only options in such cases were crowns or removable dentures. The problem with such conventional dentures, though, is that they are difficult to keep in place, making it difficult to eat hard foods such as apples or potatoes. This can cause embarrassment when eating in public. Moreover, such dentures must be taken out overnight.

However, we now have another option : dental implants. Implants have a big advantage over conventional dentures. Usually made of titanium or titanium alloy, implants actually fuse to the bone, becoming part of your body. A replacement tooth, or dental crown, or partial or full dentures can then be fixed to the implant. Such implants are very secure. This means that you can speak and eat even hard foods with complete confidence. Implants also help fill out your cheeks, which may look sunken if you lose too many teeth, making you look old. And they do not have to be removed overnight.

So, what is a dental implant? Well, it looks like a screw and acts as a tooth root (See picture). It can be used in the lower jaw, known as the *mandible*, or upper jaw, known as the maxilla. Just as a root does for a natural tooth, the implant anchors the dental crown or denture to the jaw.

Having an implant requires surgery, which usually takes around 6 months to complete. First, the dentist makes a hole in the jaw and inserts the implant, usu-

36 ● Unit 4 Dental Implants

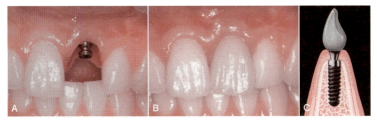

インプラントとは，歯の抜けた部分に人工歯根（インプラント）を埋め込み，その上に人工の歯冠を装着する治療のことである．その結果，失った機能（食べる，飲み込む，発音する）と形態を回復し，残っている歯とそれを支える骨を守ることができる．A：インプラントが植立されたところ，B：インプラント上部構造が装着されたところ，C：インプラントの模式図．

ally fixing a screw into the implant to prevent gum tissue or debris from your mouth getting inside. Gum tissue is then secured in place over the implant. The dentist will then wait for the implant to fuse to the bone, a process called *osseointegration*. When this is done, he will uncover the implant, attach a post (if one is not already attached) and allow the gum tissue to heal around it. Finally, he will attach the crown to the post.

Not everybody can have this done, though. You have to be in good general health and maintain good *oral hygiene*. It also helps to be young, as the bone gets weaker with age. The main *drawback* with implants is jaw joint, known as the *temporomandibular joint*, pain. The implant is more secure than a natural tooth and it has no nerves. Therefore, you can *chew* too strongly without realizing it, which will lead to pain. Moreover, the implants have to be professionally cleaned by your dentist on a regular basis.

 Coffee Break

インプラント（implant）は「死んだ組織」や「人工材料」を用いて生体の欠損を補充し，機能を回復させることをいう．移植（transplant）は「生きた組織」を他の場所に移し機能させることをいう．自分の組織を移植する場合を自家移植という．歯の場合には自家歯牙移植といい，移植免疫（非自己を排除する）の問題はないものの，供給量に限界がある．一方，他人の歯を移植することを他家歯牙移植といい，供給量に限界がないものの，移植免疫が大きな問題となる．また，動物などの歯を使う場合は異種歯牙移植といい，移植免疫はさらに大きな問題となる．

Read 1

Fast Facts : Read through the passage quickly and complete this grid. Then check your answers with a partner.

1. Losing teeth due to _____ or _____ can cause _____ problems. 2. In the past, you had to have _____ _____. 3. Unfortunately, removable dentures have to be _____ _____ overnight. 4. These days, you can choose _____ _____ instead. 5. Usually made of _____ or _____ _____, they actually _____ _____ bone. They act as a _____ _____, and can be put in the upper jaw, the _____, or the lower jaw, the _____. 6. The process by which the implant fuses with the bone is called _____. 7. To have one, you have to be in good general _____ and have good _____ _____. 8. However, implants do have some _____. 9. The main problem is pain in the _____ _____. 10. This occurs because people _____ too strongly.

Read 2

How much did you understand?

Answer true (T) or false (F) to each of these statements :
1. Losing teeth can not affect your ability to speak. (   )
2. The only options now are crowns or removable dentures. (   )
3. Conventional dentures must be taken out overnight. (   )
4. Conventional dentures are easy to keep in place. (   )
5. Implants allow you to eat even hard foods without worry. (   )
6. The dentist makes a hole in the jaw and inserts the implant. (   )
7. The lower jaw is called the temporomandibular joint. (   )

Read 3

Let's answer : Now try and answer these questions based on the text.

1. What are two things that can cause tooth loss?
2. How can tooth loss affect you?
3. Why are conventional dentures unsatisfactory?
4. What does an implant do that a conventional denture does not?
5. Why does the dentist usually fix a screw into the implant?
6. What is the final stage in the process?
7. What is the biggest problem with implants?
8. Why does this problem occur?

Listening

Word focus : Listen to this extract from the text a few times and circle the correct word in each of the sentences 1~4. 🔊 *25*

1. Usually made of titanium or titanium alloy, implants actually (refuse / fuse) to the bone, becoming (part / art) of your body.
2. A replacement tooth, or dental crown, or (part shell / partial) or full dentures can then be (fixed / fitted) to the implant.
3. Well, it looks like a (crew / screw) and acts as a tooth root.
4. Just as a root does for a natural tooth, the implant (anchors / incurs) the dental (clown / crown) or denture to the jaw.

Part 3 : Dialogue

1) Preliminary listening exercises

Keywords : Here are 10 keywords from the dialogue. Listen and number them in the order you hear them. 🔊 *26*

advantages ( ) antibiotics ( ) diabetes ( ) oral hygiene ( )
infection ( ) general health ( ) dental implant ( ) pain killers ( )
crown ( ) history of heart disease ( )

Question focus : The dentist gives the patient some information and advice. Listen and complete what the dentist says. 🔊 *27*

1. Do you have _____?
2. Do you have any history of _____ _____ or other _____ _____?
3. _____ _____ do you brush your teeth?
4. Well, I would like to _____ a dental implant.
5. Well, they _____ the tooth _____ more securely to the jaw.
6. So you can eat anything, even _____ or _____ foods.
7. It'll take around _____ months, altogether.

2) Listening

Cover the dialogue below and just listen two or three times. Finally, number these sentences in the order you hear them 1~5. 🔊 *28*

1. Sounds great. How long will it take? ( )
2. There is the risk of some pain and infection. ( )
3. How often do you see a dentist? ( )
4. Which is cheaper, an implant or ordinary dentures? ( )
5. However, we can control both with pain killers and antibiotics. ( )

3) **Activity**

Step 1 : Read the dialogue below. Use your dictionary and ask your teacher if there is anything you do not understand. When you have read and understood the dialogue, take turns reading each part with a partner. Try this : 1) Look at each line. 2) Cover each line. 3) Read each line without looking.

In the clinic : Implants

Patient : I look terrible with these three front teeth missing. Is there anything you can do?

Dentist : Do you have diabetes?

Patient : No.

Dentist : Do you have any history of heart disease or other serious illnesses?

Patient : No, my doctor says I am in good general health.

Dentist : How often do you brush your teeth?

Patient : Three times a day, after meals.

Dentist : This is your first time at this clinic. How often do you see a dentist?

Patient : Well, I have just moved here. Usually, I visit the dentist around once every three months.

Dentist : You are around 40 years old, right?

Patient : Yes, that's right. Why do you want to know?

Dentist : Well, I would like to recommend a dental implant. But you need to be in good health and maintain good oral hygiene for that.

Patient : Which is cheaper, an implant or ordinary dentures?

Dentist : Ordinary dentures.

Patient : So, what are the advantages of an implant?

Dentist : Well, they anchor the tooth crown more securely to the jaw. So you can eat anything, even hard or sticky foods.

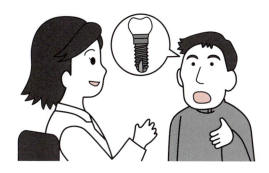

Patient : Is that all?

Dentist : No. You can also speak with confidence, as you don't have to worry about your teeth falling out!

Patient : Sounds great. How long will it take?

Dentist : It'll take around 6 months, altogether.

Patient : Will it hurt?

Dentist : There is the risk of some pain and infection. However, we can control both with pain killers and antibiotics.

Note : "visit the dentist / doctor" and "see the dentist / doctor" mean the same as "go to the dentist / doctor / hospital / clinic" in English.

Vocabulary Notes

- diabetes　糖尿病．血液の中に含まれる糖の濃度が高い状態が続き，尿の中にブドウ糖が排泄される病気．食事で摂取する糖質はブドウ糖となり，腸から吸収されて血液中に入る．このブドウ糖は脳，筋肉，肝臓などに取り込まれて，エネルギー源として役に立つ．ブドウ糖の調節はインスリンというホルモンが司るが，インスリンの機能低下により血糖がスムーズに細胞内に入らず，結果，血糖値が高くなる．
- serious illnesses　重大な病気．簡単に治癒するようなものでなく，日常生活に支障をきたし，最悪の場合には死にもつながるような疾患をさす．
- general health　全身の健康状態．健康とは，WHOによれば，食欲があり，風邪をひかず，ひどく疲れず，よく眠れるとある．
- oral　口腔．口腔は消化管の最前端で，食物を取り入れる部分で，鼻腔とならんで呼吸器の末端でもある．付属器として，歯，舌，外分泌器（唾液腺）等を備えている．
- infection　感染．微生物が宿主に侵入・定着した状態で，定着後は宿主の栄養や機能を利用しながら増殖し，宿主に何らかの病状を発症させる一連の過程．微生物が皮膚などに着いた状態は汚染といい，区別される．
- pain killers　鎮痛薬．痛みを和らげたり取り除く医薬品の総称．
- antibiotics　抗生物質．細菌の増殖を抑制したり殺したりする作用をもつ物質．

Step 2 : Now take turns playing the dentist or the patient. Your questions and answers do not have to be exactly the same as in the dialogue above.

Word stew

Can you unscramble these words?

ciiotsbinta
baiesetd
lebidnam
proometdmanbiralu
aaxllim

Micro-presentation

In a group, make a list of the advantages and disadvantages of dental implants. Then practice giving a short presentation on this topic.

Tales from the clinic

歯科インプラントは，義歯やブリッジと並ぶ補綴治療で，天然歯と遜色ない機能と審美性をもっている．しかし，生体の骨の中に金属を埋め込んで使用するため，基礎疾患をもつ患者，たとえば糖尿病などの患者では，植立にあたり，細心の注意が必要となる．また，非自己であるため，常に生体の排除機転にさらされており，感染すれば脱落への道をたどることも重要な留意点である．

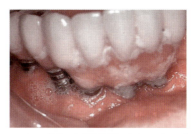

インプラント周囲炎により，インプラント体が露出している．

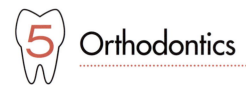

5 Orthodontics

Part 1 : Vocabulary

Some of these words are just for you : the professional dentist. If you use them to a patient, they may not understand. These words are in red, *italicized* font in the text. Some words you can use among professionals *and* to patients : these are in ordinary red font.

1) Listen and number the words in the order you hear them 1~13. 🔊 *29*

orthodontics ( ) irregular ( ) orthodontic treatment ( ) orthodontist ( )
crooked ( ) stick out ( ) crowding ( ) malocclusion ( )
plaster models ( ) appliances ( ) removable braces ( )
fixed brace ( ) retainer ( )

2)

Step 1 : Repeat these words after you hear them. 🔊 *30*
Step 2 : Study the vocabulary list by yourself for a few minutes.
Step 3 : Make groups of up to 4 students. Test each other : one student chooses an English or Japanese word at random and the other students have to guess the translation.

Note : Don't worry if you do not understand these words, even in translation. Just get used to hearing and saying them.

Vocabulary List

orthodontics	歯科矯正
irregular	乱れた，ふぞろいな
orthodontic treatment	矯正処置
orthodontist	歯科矯正医
straightening	矯正，まっすぐにする
function	機能
crooked	曲がっている
stick out	出っ張る，突出する
protrude	はみ出る，突出する
crowding	叢生
extract	抜歯する／抜歯
incorrect bite	不正咬合
malocclusion	不正咬合
plaster models	石膏模型
consultation	診察，相談
treatment plan	治療計画
appliances	装置，器具
braces	矯正装置
removable	可綴性の，取りはずしできる
fixed	固定性の
headgear	ヘッドギア
retainer	リテーナー，保定装置

Coffee Break

　歯並びが悪いことにコンプレックスを抱く人が世界的に増加している．もちろん，歯を動かすことは容易ではない．矯正治療がすべて終了するまでに2，3年以上は必要となる．しかし，とくに女性は治療後のQOLが激変し，お化粧や服の好みも変わり，行動も華やかになるとかならないとか……

3) Match the English words with their Japanese translation.

orthodontics ·   · 矯正装置

irregular ·   · 診察，相談

orthodontic treatment ·   · 矯正処置

orthodontist ·   · 歯科矯正医

straightening ·   · 出っ張る，突出する

function ·   · 機能

crooked ·   · 曲がっている

stick out ·   · 乱れた，ふぞろいな

protrude ·   · はみ出る，突出する

crowding ·   · ヘッドギア

extract ·   · 歯科矯正

incorrect bite ·   · 不正咬合

malocclusion ·   · 不正咬合

plaster models ·   · 石膏模型

consultation ·   · リテーナー，保定装置

treatment plan ·   · 治療計画

appliances ·   · 可綴性の，取りはずしできる

braces ·   · 矯正，まっすぐにする

removable ·   · 固定性の

fixed ·   · 抜歯する / 抜歯

headgear ·   · 叢生

retainer ·   · 装置，器具

4) Listen and write down the word or words you hear. 🔊 *31*

1. _____   2. _____.

3. _____   4. _____.

5. _____.

Part 2 : Reading

Note : Reading strategy

Step 1 : Just read through as quickly as you can. Do not use your dictionary.

Step 2 : Read again more slowly. Underline any words you do not know. Use your dictionary *after* you have finished reading. Do not try to memorize more than a few words at one go.

Step 3 : Read through again at normal speed.

Orthodontics

Orthodontics is a branch of dentistry that specializes in treating patients with irregular teeth. The word orthodontics comes from two Greek words : *orthos*, which means straight or proper, and *odous*, which means tooth. A dentist who specializes in orthodontic treatment is called an orthodontist. Orthodontic treatment is a way of straightening or moving teeth so that the appearance of the teeth and also their function are improved.

Patients who need orthodontic treatment will typically have some of the following problems. Crooked teeth : these not only look bad, but are also difficult to clean. People with this problem tend to have more cavities and gum problems than people with straight teeth. Some people will have teeth that stick out ; another word for this is 'protrude'. Others will suffer from crowding, which is lack of space for all the teeth to fit normally in the jaws. As a result, the teeth may be twisted or out of position. If the case involves extreme crowding, it might be necessary to extract one or more teeth. In some cases, the upper and lower jaw may not meet correctly and this can lead to an incorrect bite, which is known as *malocclusion*.

The first appointment with an orthodontist will involve a full examination, where your teeth are checked and x-rays taken. The orthodontist will also take plaster models of your teeth. After consultation, a treatment plan will be agreed on and then treatment will go ahead.

Orthodontic treatment involves the use of many types of appliances, which are called *braces*. Such braces can be either removable or fixed. Removable brac-

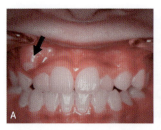 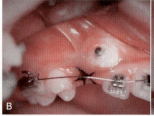 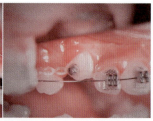

歯科矯正は，乱ぐい歯，叢生，反対咬合などの歯の配列異常をもつ患者に，ワイヤーなどを装着し，その矯正力により歯を正常な位置に移動させたり，上顎骨，下顎骨の形態変化を起こすことで，審美性や顎口腔機能を回復することを目的とする．不正咬合は多くの疾患や機能障害の原因となるので，これを取り除く矯正歯科の役割は大きい．A：犬歯（←）が萌出できない症例，B：第一小臼歯を抜歯して，犬歯の入る場所をつくり，そこへワイヤーとラバーで犬歯を移動させている（左：抜歯後，右：移動中）．

es are generally used in simple treatment and consist of a plate that can be removed from the mouth for cleaning. The plate has wires attached that are used to move the teeth. In most cases, patients having orthodontic treatment will have fixed appliances fitted. In this case, brackets and bands are attached to the teeth. A flexible wire joins all the brackets and this allows the teeth to move. Since patients are unable to remove the appliance from their mouths, it is called a fixed appliance. Brackets are made of metal and sometimes of plastic or ceramic. As well as a brace, your dentist may ask you to wear headgear in the evening or at night.

  The success of orthodontic treatment partly depends on the effort the patient puts in. This will involve attending the dental clinic regularly and following the instructions of the orthodontist as well as the dental hygienist. Patients should realize that even after treatment has finished it will be necessary to wear a retainer for a few nights a week.

Read 1

Fast Facts : Read through the passage quickly and complete this grid. Then check your answers with a partner.

1. The word _____ comes from two Greek words : '*orthos*' and '*odous*'. 2. A dentist who specializes in orthodontic treatment is called an _____. 3. The aim of orthodontic treatment is to improve the _____ of the teeth as well as their _____. 4. Teeth that are not straight are called _____. 5. If you have lack of space in your jaws, you will probably have a problem with _____. 6. An incorrect bite is known as _____. 7. After a consultation with an orthodontist, a _____ _____ will be agreed on. 8. Braces are either _____ or _____. 9. As well as a brace, you may need to wear _____ at night. 10. After the treatment, you will need to wear a _____ for a few nights a week.

Read 2

How much did you understand?

Answer true (T) or false (F) to each of these statements :
1. Orthodontics specializes in treating people with straight teeth. (   )
2. One of the aims of orthodontic treatment is to improve the function of the teeth. (   )
3. People with straight teeth tend to have more cavities than people with crooked teeth. (   )
4. In cases of extreme crowding, it will be unnecessary to extract any teeth. (   )
5. When the upper and lower teeth meet correctly, this is known as malocclusion. (   )
6. At the first appointment, the dentist will check your teeth, take x-rays and fit a brace to your teeth. (   )

49

Read 3

Let's answer : Now try and answer these questions based on the text.

1. What do the Greek words '*orthos*' and '*odous*' mean?
2. What is the technical term for an incorrect bite?
3. How many types of braces are there? What are they called?
4. What are the brackets made of?
5. What will the patient probably need to wear after the treatment is over?

Listening

Word focus : Listen to the sentences (1~5) and circle the correct words. 🔊 *32*

1. orthodontics, orthodontic treatment, orthodontist
2. crooked, crowding, malocclusion
3. appliances, brace, plate
4. removable, fixed, headgear
5. patient, orthodontist, dental hygienist

Part 3 : Dialogue

1) Preliminary listening exercises

Keywords : Here are 17 keywords from the dialogue. Listen and number them in the order you hear them. 🔊 *33*

smile (　) crooked (　) crowding (　) taken out (　) extract (　)
severity (　) adjusting (　) braces (　) removable (　) permanent (　)
sugary food (　) dental hygienist (　) lifestyle (　) hard food (　)
sticky food (　) plaque (　) retainers (　)

Question focus : A patient is asking an orthodontist about orthodontic treatment. Listen and complete the questions. 🔊 *34*

1. But I'm 25 years old. _____ _____ _____ _____ _____?
2. Would I need to _____ _____ _____ _____ _____?
3. How long _____ _____ _____ _____?
4. How often will I need _____ _____ _____ _____ _____?
5. What types of _____ _____ _____?
6. How would I need to care _____ _____ _____ _____ _____ during treatment?
7. Will braces _____ _____ _____?
8. Is _____ _____ _____?

● 51

2) Listening

Cover the dialogue below and just listen two or three times. Finally, number these sentences in the order you hear them. 🔊 *35*

1. If crowding is a problem, it might be necessary to extract some teeth in order to make space. ( )
2. Your braces will need adjusting every 6 to 8 weeks. ( )
3. Basically, there are two types : removable and permanent. ( )
4. Orthodontic treatment can be successful at any age. It is never too late to have treatment. ( )
5. You will need to make some small changes. ( )
6. You would also need to reduce the amount of sugary food and drinks you consume. ( )
7. In general, most patients can be treated within two years. ( )

3) Activity

Step 1 : Read the dialogue below. Use your dictionary and ask your teacher if there is anything you do not understand. When you have read and understood the dialogue, take turns reading each part with a partner. Try this : 1) Look at each line. 2) Cover each line. 3) Read each line without looking.

In the clinic : Orthodontics

Patient : I'd like to ask some questions about orthodontic treatment.
Dentist : What would you like to know?
Patient : I'm not happy with my smile. Some of my teeth are crooked. My regular dentist said I have a problem with crowding. But I'm 25 years old. Can I have orthodontic treatment?
Dentist : Yes. Orthodontic treatment can be successful at any age. It is never too late to have treatment.
Patient : Would I need to have any teeth taken out?
Dentist : If crowding is a problem, it might be necessary to extract some teeth in order to make space. Sometimes space can be created by other forms of treatment.
Patient : How long will the treatment take?
Dentist : It depends on the severity of the problem. In general, most patients can be treated within two years.
Patient : How often will I need to visit the dental clinic?
Dentist : Your braces will need adjusting every 6 to 8 weeks. You would probably need to visit us every two months.
Patient : What types of braces are available?
Dentist : Basically, there are two types : removable and permanent. Removable braces can be taken out for cleaning. Permanent braces are fixed to the teeth and cannot be taken out for cleaning.
Patient : How would I need to care for my teeth and braces during treatment?

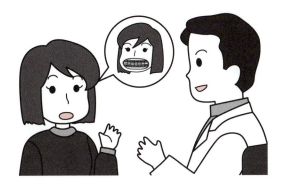

Dentist : During orthodontic treatment, you would need to take extra care of your teeth. You need to brush your teeth and the braces very carefully. You would also need to reduce the amount of sugary food and drinks you consume. And you would need to visit the dental hygienist regularly for advice on brushing.

Patient : Will braces change my lifestyle?

Dentist : You will need to make some small changes. For example, you will need to avoid hard and sticky foods that might damage your braces. Also it is very important to keep your braces and teeth clean and free of plaque.

Patient : Is orthodontic treatment permanent?

Dentist : It is probable that your teeth will move over time. So we advise you to wear retainers at night once or twice a week after treatment has finished.

Vocabulary Note
- permanent　永久の，常置の
- plaque　プラーク，歯垢

Step 2 : Now take turns playing the dentist or the patient. Your questions and answers do not have to be exactly the same as in the dialogue above.

Word stew

Can you unscramble these words?

dtorhtooncsi
dcrkeoo
wdngcrio
lamnioccosul
sbreac

Tales from the clinic

　矯正治療によって,「機能」と「見た目」の2つの問題を解決することができる.機能的なメリットとしては,唇がスムーズに閉じやすくなったり,ブラッシングがしやすくなるため,虫歯や歯周病をはじめ,口の中のトラブルが起こりにくくなり,噛み合わせがよくなることで,消化器官を正常に機能させることができる.「見た目」のメリットも大きく,歯並びがキレイになることで口元がすっきりと美しくなり,コンプレックスも解消し,人生に積極的になったり,性格まで明るくなることもまれではない.

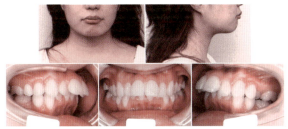

矯正前(上顎前突と深い咬み合わせがみられる)

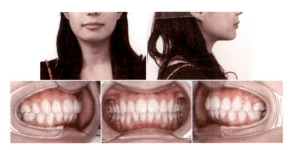

矯正後(問題点はほぼ解決された)

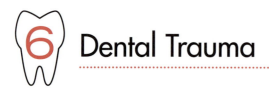

6 Dental Trauma

Part 1 : Vocabulary

Some of these words are just for you : the professional dentist. If you use them to a patient, they may not understand. These words are in red, *italicized* font in the text. Some words you can use among professionals and to patients : these are in ordinary red font.

1) Listen and number the words in the order you hear them 1~15. 🔊 *36*

   trauma ( ) cheeks ( ) jawbones ( ) fractured ( ) extrusion ( )
   avulsed ( ) swollen ( ) painful ( ) bloody ( ) knocked out ( )
   socket ( ) crown ( ) root ( ) saline ( ) moist ( )

2)

Step 1 : Repeat these words after you hear them. 🔊 *37*

Step 2 : Study the vocabulary list by yourself for a few minutes.

Step 3 : Make groups of up to 4 students. Test each other : one student chooses an English or Japanese word at random and the other students have to guess the translation.

Note : Don't worry if you do not understand these words, even in translation. Just get used to hearing and saying them.

Vocabulary List

trauma	外傷	swollen	腫れた
cheeks	頬	painful	痛い，有痛性の
jawbones	顎骨	bloody	出血している，観血的な
chipped	欠けた	cold compress	冷湿布
fractured	折れた	permanent tooth	永久歯
extrusion	挺出，突出	crown	クラウン，歯冠
loosened	緩んだ	root	歯根
intrusion	嵌入，侵入	saline	生理食塩水
knocked out	たたいて抜けた	moist	湿った，湿気のある
socket	歯槽，抜歯窩	reimplanted	再植された
avulsed	脱臼した，引き離された（捻除）	stitches	縫合

3) Match the English words with their Japanese translation.

trauma ·   · 生理食塩水
jawbones ·   · 嵌入，侵入
fractured ·   · 顎骨
extrusion ·   · 歯槽，抜歯窩
loosened ·   · 挺出，突出
intrusion ·   · 緩んだ
knocked out ·   · 再植された
socket ·   · 湿った，湿気のある
avulsed ·   · 脱臼した，引き離された（捻除）
swollen ·   · 腫れた
bloody ·   · 出血している，観血的な
saline ·   · 折れた
moist ·   · 外傷
reimplanted ·   · たたいて抜けた

4) Listen and write down the word or words you hear. 🔊 *38*

1. _____.   2. _____.
3. _____.   4. _____.
5. _____.

● 57

Part 2 : Reading

Note : Reading strategy

Step 1 : Just read through as quickly as you can. Do not use your dictionary.

Step 2 : Read again more slowly. Underline any words you do not know. Use your dictionary *after* you have finished reading. Do not try to memorize more than a few words at one go.

Step 3 : Read through again at normal speed.

Dental Trauma

Dental trauma usually involves injury to the mouth, including the teeth, lips, gums, tongue, cheeks and jawbones. The most common type of dental trauma is a broken or knocked-out tooth.

Dental trauma usually occurs as a result of accidents. These include car crashes, and accidents involving motor bikes or bicycles. It also occurs as a result of tripping or slipping. Dental trauma is also particularly common in contact sports such as ice hockey, football, and rugby. Street fights and physical assaults are also common causes of dental trauma.

As a result of dental trauma, teeth may be chipped, cracked or broken. The technical term for broken is *fractured*. In some cases, teeth may have been pushed out of position. This is known as *extrusion*. Teeth may have been loosened by the impact of the accident, which is known as *concussion*. Teeth may also have been pushed up into the jaw. This is known as *intrusion*. In extreme cases, a tooth may have been knocked out of its socket. This is known as an *avulsed* tooth. In many cases, the oral tissues will have been injured and consequently will be swollen, painful and bloody.

How is dental trauma treated? If a patient has a swollen lip, the swelling can be reduced by applying a cold compress or ice pack. Bleeding can be stopped by applying pressure to the wound using a gauze pad. Patients with deep cuts will require stitches. Treatment of a broken tooth will depend on the type of injury. For a tooth that has been knocked out of its *socket*, it is important to act quickly. First, search the area around where the injury took place so that you can find the

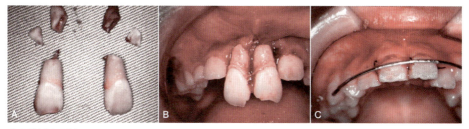

歯の破折と再植

　歯が破折，脱臼してしまっても状態がよければ，再植することができる．再植とは，抜けてしまった歯を元の位置に戻して，固定し，再び機能させる治療のことである．この症例では，前歯2本が完全に脱臼してしまい，根尖で破折していた（A）．消毒後，折れた歯根尖は使わず，再植（B），固定した（C）．

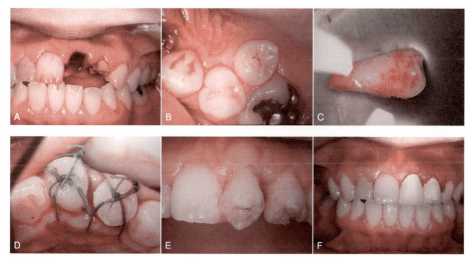

歯の移植

　移植とは，歯の抜けた部分（A）に自分のいらない歯（B）を抜歯（C）して，歯の抜けたところに埋め込み固定し（D），生体に生着させる（E）．その後，審美性を考慮した治療を行い，機能させる治療のことである（F）．この症例は，たまたま上顎に2本の転移歯（B）があり，移植を行うことができた．

tooth. Remember that a knocked-out permanent tooth will die unless it is returned to the socket as quickly as possible. When you pick up the tooth, make sure you pick it up by the crown and do not touch the root. Rinse the tooth in cold water to remove any dirt. Do not scrub it with soap or toothpaste. Put the tooth back into the socket and bite down on it. If this is done in the first 20 minutes, there is a 90 percent chance of tooth survival. Thirty or 60 minutes cuts the survival rate to 75 percent. If it does not easily go back into the socket, you should keep it in your mouth until you reach the dental clinic. If it is not possible to put your tooth back into your mouth immediately, put it in milk or *saline*. It is important to keep the tooth moist. You should aim to bring the patient and the tooth to the dental clinic within 30 minutes of the accident. If all of the above are done, there is a possibility that a permanent tooth that has been knocked out can be successfully *reimplanted*.

Read 1

Fast Facts : Read through the passage quickly and complete this grid. Then check your answers with a partner.

1. Dental trauma usually occurs as a result of _____. 2. Dental trauma is particularly common in _____ sports. 3. The technical term for a broken tooth is a _____ tooth. 4. A tooth that has been knocked out is called an _____ tooth. 5. People with dental trauma will probably have _____ lips. 6. Swelling can be reduced by applying a _____ _____. 7. When a tooth has been knocked out of its socket, it is important to act _____. 8. When you pick up a knocked-out tooth, make sure you pick it up by the _____. 9. Do not touch the _____. 10. It is important to keep the tooth _____.

60 ● Unit 6 Dental Trauma

Read 2

How much did you understand?

Answer true (T) or false (F) to each of these statements.

1. When teeth are pushed out of position, this is known as fractured. ( )
2. When teeth are loosened by the impact of the accident, this is known as concussion. ( )
3. When a tooth has been knocked out of its socket, this is known as an avulsed tooth. ( )
4. Bleeding can be stopped by applying a cold compress. ( )
5. If a knocked-out tooth is put back into its socket in the first 20 minutes, there is a 90 percent chance of tooth survival. ( )
6. If a knocked-out tooth is put back into its socket in 30 to 60 minutes, there is a 50 percent chance of tooth survival. ( )
7. It's okay to keep a knocked-out tooth in cold water. ( )
8. You should try to bring the patient and the tooth to the dental clinic within three hours. ( )

Read 3

Let's answer : Now try and answer these questions based on the text.

1. In what kind of sports is dental trauma particularly common?
2. What is the technical term for a knocked-out tooth?
3. When would a patient require stitches?
4. If a knocked-out tooth is not returned to its socket quickly, what will happen to it?
5. If a knocked-out tooth cannot be put back into the socket, where should it be kept?

Listening

Technical term focus : Listen and complete the sentences with the correct technical terms. 🔊 *39*

1. The technical term for broken is _____.
2. In some cases, teeth may have been pushed out of position. This is known as _____.
3. As a result of an accident, teeth may have been loosened. This is known as _____.
4. Teeth may also have been pushed up into the jaw. This is known as _____.
5. In extreme cases, a tooth may have been knocked out of its socket. This is known as an _____ tooth.

☕ *Coffee Break*

　歯の外傷は，子どもやスポーツ選手など活発な動きをする人たちに起こりやすい．正常な歯が折れるときは，横に割れることが多いが，う蝕などで歯の神経（歯髄）を除去してしまうと，縦に折れることが多い．これは，生竹と乾燥した死竹の関係によく似ている．現在，多くのスポーツでマウスガードの装着がみられるが，これは歯の外傷の予防に非常に有効な手段であり，高校性のラグビー選手はマウスガードの装着が義務づけられている．

Part 3 : Dialogue

1) Preliminary listening exercises

Keywords : Here are 16 keywords from the dialogue. Listen and number them in the order you hear them. 🔊 *40*

fracture (　) knock out (　) accident (　) sports injury (　) lips (　)
swelling (　) bleeding (　) in a state of shock (　) pass out (　)
lost consciousness (　) accident and emergency unit (　) reimplant (　)
moist (　) saliva (　) scrub (　) rinse (　)

Question focus : A dental student is asking a teacher some questions about dental trauma. Listen and complete the questions. 🔊 *41*

1. You said people sometimes fracture or knock out a tooth. _____ _____ _____ _____ _____ ?
2. As well as the problem with their tooth, will _____ _____ _____ _____ _____ as a result of the fall?
3. How will the patient _____ _____ _____ _____ _____ ?
4. I heard that sometimes patients pass out. What _____ _____ _____ in that case?
5. When you take the patient to the dental clinic for treatment, _____ _____ _____ _____ ?
6. What should you do with a _____ _____ _____ _____ _____ _____ ?
7. What is the best place to _____ _____ _____ _____ ?
8. What should you do _____ _____ _____ _____ _____ ?

2) Listening

Cover the dialogue below and just listen two or three times. Finally, number these sentences in the order you hear them 1~8. 🔊 *42*

1. If a patient has lost consciousness, he or she should be taken immediately to the nearest accident and emergency unit. ( )
2. Yes. In many cases they will have damage to the lips, swelling and bleeding. ( )
3. It may be possible to reimplant it, so keep it warm and moist in saliva or warm milk. ( )
4. In the patient's own mouth, between the cheek and the lower lip. ( )
5. In most cases, because of a fall or some kind of an accident, such as a car accident or a sports injury. ( )
6. One thing to remember is that you should bring any pieces of the tooth with you. ( )
7. Never scrub it. Just rinse it briefly under cold water. ( )
8. Well, it depends on the person. In the beginning, the patient may not feel a lot of pain. But some patients might be in a state of shock. ( )

3) Activity

Step 1 : Read the dialogue below. Use your dictionary and ask your teacher if there is anything you do not understand. When you have read and understood the dialogue, take turns reading each part with a partner. Try this : 1. Look at each line. 2) Cover each line. 3) Read each line without looking.

A dental student is asking a teacher some questions about dental trauma.

Student : Excuse me, I have a question.

Dentist : Yes, of course. What would you like to know?

Student : You said people sometimes fracture or knock out a tooth. How does that usually happen?

Dentist : In most cases, because of a fall or some kind of an accident, such as a car accident or a sports injury.

Student : As well as the problem with their tooth, will patients have any other problems as a result of the fall?

Dentist : Yes. In many cases, they will have damage to the lips, swelling and bleeding.

Student : How will the patient feel immediately after the accident?

Dentist : Well, it depends on the person. In the beginning, the patient may not feel a lot of pain. But some patients might be in a state of shock.

Student : I heard that sometimes patients pass out. What should be done in that case?

Dentist : If a patient has lost consciousness, he or she should be taken immediately to the nearest accident and emergency unit.

Student : When you take the patient to the dental clinic for treatment, what should you do?

Dentist : One thing to remember is that you should bring any pieces of the tooth with you.

Student : What should you do with a tooth that has been knocked out?

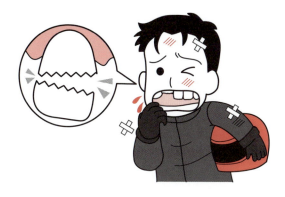

Dentist : It may be possible to reimplant it, so keep it warm and moist in saliva or warm milk.
Student : What is the best place to keep a knocked out tooth?
Dentist : In the patient's own mouth, between the cheek and the lower lip.
Student : What should you do if the tooth is dirty?
Dentist : Never scrub it. Just rinse it briefly under cold water.
Student : Thank you.

Vocabulary Notes

- shock　ショック．急激に全身性に起こる末梢血液循環障害で，激しい疼痛などで顔面が蒼白となり，冷汗をかき，脈は速いが弱くなり，呼吸不全等を起こす．
- pass out　意識を失う，気絶する
- lose consciousness　意識を失う，気絶する
- saliva　唾液

Step 2 : Now take turns playing the dentist or the patient. Your questions and answers do not have to be exactly the same as in the dialogue above.

Word stew

Can you unscramble these words?

aamurt
tdfrraecu
wnseoll
kkdoecn tuo
mieranlpt

Tales from the clinic

　歯が欠損した場所は，義歯，ブリッジそしてインプラントにより機能を回復する．しかしそれ以前に，もし歯が折れたり脱臼してしまっても，それを元の場所に戻し（再植），機能させることができればそれに越したことはない．また，折れた歯が使えなくなってしまっても，他に使える歯（親知らずや過剰歯）を移植して使うことができれば，前述の3つの治療法に勝ると考えられる．しかし，その成否は歯の周囲に存在する歯根膜という軟組織をいかに温存できるかにかかっている．感染している場合はもちろんうまくいかない．

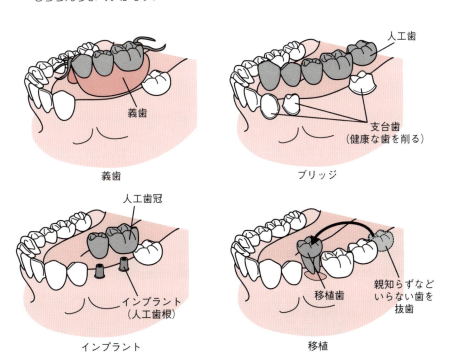

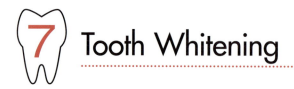

Tooth Whitening

Part 1 : Vocabulary

Some of these words are just for you : the professional dentist. If you use them to a patient, they may not understand. These words are in red, *italicized* font in the text. Some words you can use among professionals *and* to patients : these are in ordinary red font.

1) Listen and number the words in the order you hear them 1~15. 🔊 *43*

   cosmetic dentistry (　) discoloration (　) enamel (　) stained (　)
   tetracycline (　) in-office bleaching (　) chairside bleaching (　)
   at-home bleaching (　) over-the-counter (　) mouth tray (　)
   bleaching gel (　) side effects (　) sensitivity (　) irritation (　)
   hydrogen peroxide (　)

2)

Step 1 : Repeat these words after you hear them. 🔊 *44*

Step 2 : Study the vocabulary list by yourself for a few minutes.

Step 3 : Make groups of up to 4 students. Test each other : one student chooses an English or Japanese word at random and the other students have to guess the translation.

Note : Don't worry if you do not understand these words, even in translation. Just get used to hearing and saying them.

Vocabulary List

cosmetic dentistry 審美歯科	mineral structure of the tooth 歯のミネラル構造
discoloration 変色	stained 着色された，汚れた
enamel エナメル質	antibiotic medicines 抗菌性の内服薬
in-office bleaching オフィスブリーチング	tetracycline テトラサイクリン
chairside bleaching チェアサイドブリーチング	dissatisfied 不満な
at-home bleaching ホームブリーチング	apply a gel to a patient's teeth 患者の歯にジェルをぬる
over-the-counter 処方箋なしで	custom-made 注文品の
mouth tray マウストレー	rubber dam ラバーダム
bleaching gel ブリーチングジェル	protective gel 保護ジェル
side effects 副作用	prescribe 処方する
sensitivity 知覚過敏，敏感性	instructions 指示書，説明書
hydrogen peroxide 過酸化水素	gingival irritation 歯肉刺激
tooth color 歯色	relapse 後戻り，後戻りする

3) Match the English words with their Japanese translation.

cosmetic dentistry ·	· 処方する
discoloration ·	· エナメル質
enamel ·	· 審美歯科
mouth tray ·	· 着色された，汚れた
hydrogen peroxide ·	· 変色
stained ·	· 過酸化水素
protective gel ·	· 保護ジェル
prescribe ·	· 歯肉刺激
gingival irritation ·	· マウストレー

4) Listen and write down the word or words you hear. 🔊 *45*

1. _____. 2. _____.
3. _____. 4. _____.
5. _____.

● 69

Part 2 : Reading

Note : Reading strategy

Step 1 : Just read through as quickly as you can. Do not use your dictionary.

Step 2 : Read again more slowly. Underline any words you do not know. Use your dictionary *after* you have finished reading. Do not try to memorize more than a few words at one go.

Step 3 : Read through again at normal speed.

Tooth Whitening

More and more people want whiter and brighter smiles. In the United States, 34 percent of the adult population reported that they are dissatisfied with their present tooth color. In the UK, up to 100,000 people a year have some type of tooth whitening treatment. This is ten times more than 5 years ago. With this level of demand, cosmetic dentistry is becoming increasingly important for many dentists.

What causes tooth *discoloration*? As a person gets older, their teeth become darker because of changes in the mineral structure of the tooth, as the enamel becomes less porous. Teeth are also stained by smoking and drinking tea, coffee and red wine. Additionally, teeth can be stained as a result of taking antibiotic medicines such as tetracycline.

If you are dissatisfied with your smile and want whiter teeth, what options are available to you? There are three main ways you can get whiter teeth. Firstly, in-office bleaching. In this case, a whitening product is applied to the patient's teeth by a dentist in the dental clinic. This is also called chairside bleaching. Secondly, at-home bleaching, where the dentist provides a whitening product and custom-made tray for the patient to use at home. Another option is whitening products that can be bought in a drug store. They are known as over-the-counter (OTC) products.

In-office whitening is done completely in the dental office. The dentist will use a whitening product containing *hydrogen peroxide* in concentrations ranging from 15 to 30 percent. Sometimes a light or laser is used to accelerate the whitening

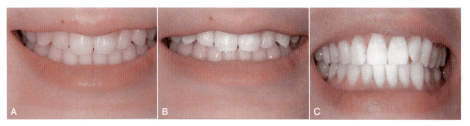

ホワイトニング（ブリーチング）とは，表面の汚れを落とすクリーニングとは異なり，歯そのものを白くするケアのことである．着色している歯の表面に過酸化水素を含むホワイトニング剤を塗って歯の色を白くしていく漂白方法である．過酸化水素は光や熱で分解されるとフリーラジカルを発生し，このフリーラジカルが着色の原因の有機物質を分解する．A：ホワイトニング前，B：上顎歯のみホワイトニング後，C：上下顎歯ホワイトニング後．

process. Before the whitening products can be applied, the dentist uses a rubber dam or protective gel to protect the gum *tissues*. The procedure is usually completed in about one hour and will require three visits on average to a dental clinic. In-office bleaching lightens teeth rapidly, but the procedure is more time-consuming for the dentist, costs more for the patient and the degree of tooth whitening is usually less than that accomplished with at-home whitening agents used in a tray.

With at-home bleaching, the dentist will make a special mouth tray that fits your teeth exactly. Your dentist will also prescribe a bleaching gel, as well as provide instructions on how to put the gel in the mouth tray. You will need to wear the mouth tray for between 30 minutes and an hour each day for two to four weeks. Your teeth should start to look whiter after a week.

Are there any side effects? Generally, the products and the procedures involved in tooth whitening are safe, but some problems have been reported. For example, mild-to-moderate tooth *sensitivity* occurs in as much as 60 percent of cases in the early stages of bleaching treatment. In addition, some people report *gingival irritation*. It is also important to remember that after treatment, your teeth will gradually begin to return to their original color, a process that is known as relapse.

Read 1

Fast Facts : Read through the passage quickly and complete this grid. Then check your answers with a partner.

1. Nowadays, lots of people are _____ with their tooth color. 2. Consequently, _____ dentistry is becoming a major part of many dentists' work. 3. _____ of your teeth is caused by changes in the mineral structure, as the enamel becomes less porous. 4. Also teeth can be _____ by smoking, and drinking tea, coffee and red wine. 5. Another word for in-office bleaching is _____ bleaching. 6. Whitening products bought in a drug store are called _____ products. 7. For at-home whitening, the dentist will make a special mouth _____ that fits your teeth exactly. 8. The dentist will also _____ a bleaching gel. 9. After bleaching, it is not unusual to experience mild-to-moderate tooth _____. 10. Some people also experience gingival _____.

Read 2

How much did you understand?
Answer true (T) or false (F) to each of these statements :

1. In the United States, about one third of adults are not happy with the color of their teeth. (　)
2. The market for cosmetic dentistry in the UK is shrinking. (　)
3. As people get older, their teeth get lighter. (　)
4. In-office bleaching and chairside bleaching are the same. (　)
5. For at-home bleaching, the dentist will provide over-the-counter products. (　)
6. For in-office bleaching, whitening products containing levels of hydrogen peroxide between 20 to 30 percent are used. (　)
7. Dentists use lights and lasers to speed up the bleaching process. (　)

8. Gum tissues are protected by a rubber dam. ( )
9. For at-home bleaching, patients wear a mouth tray every day. ( )
10. More than half of patients said they experienced tooth sensitivity. ( )

Read 3

Let's answer : Now try and answer these questions based on the text.

1. How many people had tooth whitening treatment in the UK five years ago?
2. As people get older, what happens to the enamel of their teeth?
3. How many whitening treatments are mentioned? What are they?
4. Which type of treatment costs the most?
5. For at-home bleaching, where do patients put the gel?
6. For at-home bleaching, how long do patients wear a mouth tray each day?
7. How many side effects are mentioned? What are they?

Coffee Break

　白はあらゆる可視光線を乱反射する色である．白は何色かというと，「透明」というのが正解である．たとえば透明なガラスをやすりで削れば表面に凹凸ができて，白くみえるようになる．しかし，そこに水を流せば再び透明となる．ちなみに可視光線では，最も波長が長いのが赤外線で温かさを与える．最も短いのは紫外線で，それよりも短いものは目にみえず，エックス線では物質を透過する性質をもつようになる．いずれにせよ，白色にしようとする場合には，なんらかの代償があることを忘れてはならない．

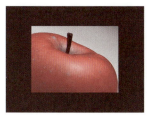
リンゴ

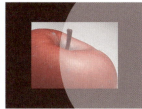
リンゴにすりガラスをかぶせると白くみえる．

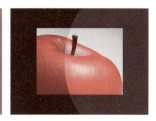
すりガラスに水を流せば透明になる．

Listening

Number focus : Listen to these 7 sentences from the text and fill in the blanks with numbers. 🔊 *46*

1. In the United States, _____ percent of the adult population reported that they are dissatisfied with their present tooth color.
2. In the UK, up to _____ people a year have some type of tooth whitening treatment.
3. This is _____ times more than _____ years ago.
4. The dentist will use a whitening product containing hydrogen peroxide in concentrations ranging from _____ to _____ percent.
5. The procedure is usually completed in about _____ hour and will require _____ visits on average to a dental clinic.
6. You will need to wear the mouth tray for between _____ minutes and an hour each day for _____ to _____ weeks.
7. For example, mild-to-moderate tooth sensitivity occurs in as much as _____ percent of cases in the early stages of bleaching treatment.

Part 3 : Dialogue

1) Preliminary listening exercises

Keywords : Here are 15 keywords from the dialogue. Listen and number them in the order you hear them. 🔊 *47*

stained ( ) treatment ( ) mouth tray ( ) prescribe ( )
hydrogen peroxide ( ) sensitivity ( ) side effect ( ) gums ( ) teeth ( )
sensitive ( ) whiter ( ) brush ( ) dental floss ( ) dental hygienist ( )
maintenance ( )

Question focus : The patient asks six questions. Listen and complete the questions. 🔊 *48*

1. _____ _____ _____ _____ _____ in-office bleaching and at-home bleaching?
2. Is the _____ _____ ?
3. Are there _____ _____ _____ ?
4. How much _____ _____ _____ _____ ?
5. How long _____ _____ _____ _____ _____ ?
6. _____ _____ _____ it cost?

2) Listening

Cover the dialogue below and just listen two or three times. Finally, number these sentences in the order you hear them 1~7. 🔊 *49*

1. They are often called OTC bleaching products. ( )
2. How can I help you today? ( )
3. You should brush twice a day, and use dental floss. ( )
4. No, it's not painful. ( )
5. It's also a good idea to come back here for maintenance every six months. ( )
6. Your teeth should become several shades lighter. ( )
7. As I said, your gums and teeth might become a little sensitive. ( )

3) Activity

Step 1 : Read the dialogue below. Use your dictionary and ask your teacher if there is anything you do not understand. When you have read and understood the dialogue, take turns reading each part with a partner. Try this : 1) Look at each line. 2) Cover each line. 3) Read each line without looking.

In the clinic : A dentist and a patient are talking about tooth whitening options.

Dentist : How can I help you today?

Patient : My teeth are really stained. I'd like to have whiter teeth.

Dentist : Well, there are several options. You can have treatment here in this dental office. It's called in-office bleaching or sometimes chairside bleaching. Or I can give you a whitening kit to use at home consisting of a mouth tray and a whitening product. That's called at-home bleaching. There are also some whitening products that you can buy over the counter. They are often called OTC bleaching products. But these products aren't very effective because they only contain very weak amounts of hydrogen peroxide.

Patient : What are the differences between in-office bleaching and at-home bleaching?

Dentist : If you have in-office bleaching, all the treatment will be done here. I will use a laser to heat the bleach. This will make the reaction go faster. With the at-home whitening kit, I will make a special mouth tray that will fit your teeth exactly. At home, you will put bleaching gel in the tray and wear it for a short time every day.

Patient : Is the treatment painful?

Dentist : No, it's not painful. But it is usual to feel some slight sensitivity after the treatment.

Patient : Are there any side effects?

Dentist : As I said, your gums and teeth might become a little sensitive. But that will be temporary. There are no long-term, harmful effects.

Patient : How much whiter will my teeth get?

Dentist : Well, it varies. Your teeth should become several shades lighter.

Patient : How long will my teeth stay white?

Dentist : It will depend on your lifestyle. If you drink a lot of coffee, tea and red wine, your teeth will get stained again. This is called relapse. But if you take care of your teeth, they will stay white longer. You should brush twice a day, and use dental floss. And you should see a dental hygienist regularly. It's also a good idea to come back here for maintenance every six months.

Patient : How much does it cost?

Dentist : Over-the-counter products will cost from 10 to 100 dollars. And an at-home bleaching kit will cost from 100 to 400 dollars. In-office bleaching will cost 650 dollars a visit.

Patient : I see. Thank you for the information.

Step 2 : Now take turns playing the dentist or the patient. Your questions and answers do not have to be exactly the same as in the dialogue above.

Vocabulary Notes
- shades　シェード，シェードガイド
- maintenance　メインテナンス

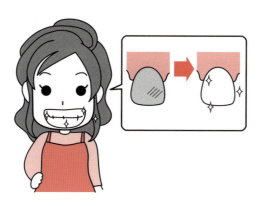

Word stew

Can you unscramble these words?

twhinegni
ssnettiiivy
edsi ffctees
rpscebeir
detsnai

Tales from the clinic

　ホワイトニングは，審美歯科の一分野であり，広義の意味では「歯を白くすること」すべてを指している．たとえば歯のクリーニング（PMTC）から始まり，ブリーチング，マニキュア，ダイレクトボンディング，ラミネートベニヤ，セラミッククラウンまで，すべてをホワイトニングということができる．狭義の意味ではいわゆる「ブリーチング（歯の漂白）」のことを指し，現在一般に使用されているホワイトニングはこのブリーチングのことを指すことが多い．ホワイトニング（いわゆるブリーチング）は，過酸化水素が分解する際に発生するヒドロキシラジカルやヒドロペルオキシラジカルなどのフリーラジカルが，歯の着色有機質の二重結合部分を切断し，低分子化することにより起こる「無色化」により，歯の明度を上げ，白くする方法である．ホワイトニングには歯科医院内で行う「オフィスホワイトニング」と，自宅で行う「ホームホワイトニング」，その中間の「アシステッドホワイトニング」，神経のない歯に対して行う「ウォーキングブリーチ」などがある．

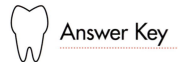

Answer Key

1. Your First Set of Teeth

Part 1 : Vocabulary

1) primary (6) deciduous (3) permanent (8) baby (2) crown (5) erupt (9) shed (12) decay (13) pacifier (1) spit out (11) rinse (10) nursing mouth syndrome (7) formula (4)

4) 1. deciduous 2. eruption 3. permanent 4. pacifier 5. primary

Read 1
1. primary / deciduous, deciduous / primary 2. permanent 3. baby 4. 6 months 5. 3 years 6. 6 years 7. 12 years 8. eating, language, place 9. affect 10. sugary liquids

Read 2
1. F 2. F 3. T 4. T 5. F 6. T 7. F

Read 3
1. jaw needs time to grow large enough 2. language, keep place for permanent teeth 3. only temporary 4. make sure the baby doesn't fall asleep with a bottle in its mouth 5. wipe baby's mouth with wet cloth

Listening
1. 20 2. 3 years 3. 6 4. 12 5. 32

Part 3 : Dialogue
Keywords
erupt (4) fall out (8) tooth decay (10) avoid (11) wipe (9) gums (2) wet cloth (5) feeding (12) brush (1) meals (3) spit out (6) rinse (7)

Question Focus
1. How long 2. Why is 3. How should 4. Should I 5. What should

2) Listening
1. (4) 2. (5) 3. (3) 4. (2) 5. (1)

Word stew
primary deciduous crown erupt decay

● 79

2. Keeping Your Teeth Looking Nice

Part 1 : Vocabulary

1) saliva (4) inflammation (5) tartar (8) calculus (6) plaque (9) bulimia (2) floss (10) colonize (11) soft-bristled (7) calcify (1) stroke (12) species (3)

4) 1. inflammation 2. bulimia 3. tartar 4. colonize 5. calcify

Read 1

1. brushing, flossing 2. plaque 3. minutes 4. saliva, sticky layer, colonized, calcify, calculus, tartar 5. brushing 6. irritate 7. floss, interdental 8. diet 9. snacking 10. bulimia

Read 2

1. T 2. F 3. F 4. T 5. T 6. F 7. T

Read 3

1. 45 degrees 2. because it might irritate gums 3. the chewing, inner and outer surfaces 4. the tip of the brush 5. your tongue 6. toward your gums 7. snap into the gums 8. toward the tip of the tooth

Listening

1. forty-five 2. Reaching 3. up-down 4. remove 5. repeat 6. interdental

Part 3 : Dialogue

Keywords

buildup (3) fluoride (9) bow-type (1) smelling (7) hard-bristled (5) angle (8) irritate (4) pairs (6) plaque (2)

Question focus

1. more carefully 2. You should 3. hold 4. back, forth 5. Don't brush 6. I recommend 7. Slide 8. back, forth

2) Listening

1. (5) 2. (3) 3. (1) 4. (6) 5. (4) 6. (2)

Word stew

buildup angle colonize calculus species

3. Tooth Decay

Part 1 : Vocabulary

1) enamel (6) debris (8) porous (3) virulence factors (11) caries (5) accumulate (12) filling (7) dentin (1) carbohydrates (9) consult (2) nerve (13) dental hygiene (10) tooth decay (4)

4) 1. porous 2. enamel 3. dentin 4. virulence 5. accumulate

Read 1
1. filling, tooth decay 2. caries 3. bacteria, *Mutans streptococcus* 4. virulence factors 5. adhere 6. acid 7. carbohydrates 8. acid 9. tissue, pulp 10. consult 11. porous

Read 2
1. F 2. T 3. T 4. F 5. F 6. T 7. F

Read 3
1. we did not understand how tooth decay works. 2. adheres to teeth, produces more acid than other bacteria, can live in that acid. 3. people don't clean their teeth, snacking, diet rich in carbohydrates. 4. through cracks in enamel 5. because nerves are in the innermost tissue, the pulp.

Listening
1. caries 2. virulence 3. adhere 4. higher 5. rich in

Part 3 : Dialogue
Key Words
interdental (4) pulp (7) checkup (1) bacteria (5) tooth decay (2) hygiene (8) pain (9) snacking (6) diet (10) floss (3) fluoride (11)

Question Focus
1. bring, in 2. getting 3. reached, pulp 4. cause, tooth decay 5. fluoride 6. floss, interdental 7. diet, hygiene

2) Listening
1. (4) 2. (1) 3. (3) 4. (5) 5. (2)

Word stew
debris caries virulence rot tissue

4. Dental Implants

Part 1 : Vocabulary

1) alloy (6) esthetic (7) titanium (11) mandible (1) trauma (10) crown (3) osseointegration (9) maxilla (5) removable dentures (13) anchor (2) temporomandibular joint (8) dental implant (12) partial dentures (4)

4) 1. temporomandibular 2. anchor 3. osseointegration 4. alloy 5. esthetic

Read 1

1. disease / trauma, trauma / disease, esthetic 2. removable dentures 3. taken out 4. dental implants 5. titanium, titanium alloy, fuse to, tooth root, maxilla, mandible 6. osseointegration 7. health, oral hygiene 8. drawbacks 9. temporomandibular joint 10. chew

Read 2

1. F 2. F 3. T 4. F 5. T 6. T 7. F

Read 3

1. disease, trauma 2. esthetic problems, ability to eat / speak 3. difficult to keep in place, difficult to eat hard foods, must take out at night 4. fuse to bone (osseointegration) 5. to prevent gum tissue or debris getting inside 6. attach crown to post 7. temporomandibular joint pain 8. chewing too strongly

Listening

1. fuse, part 2. partial, fixed 3. screw 4. anchors, crown

Part 3 : Dialogue

Keywords

advantages (10) antibiotics (5) diabetes (1) oral hygiene (3) infection (7) general health (4) dental implant (9) pain killers (2) crown (6) history of heart disease (8)

Question focus

1. diabetes 2. heart disease, serious illnesses 3. How often 4. recommend 5. anchor, crown 6. hard, sticky 7. 6

2) Listening

1. (3) 2. (4) 3. (1) 4. (2) 5. (5)

Word stew

antibiotics diabetes mandible temporomandibular maxilla

5. Orthodontics

Part 1 : Vocabulary

1) orthodontics (10) irregular (7) orthodontic treatment (11) orthodontist (2) crooked (6) stick out (4) crowding (8) malocclusion (9) plaster models (12) appliances (3) removable braces (13) fixed brace (1) retainer (5)

4) 1. crowding 2. malocclusion 3. treatment plan 4. braces 5. retainer

Read 1

1. orthodontics 2. orthodontist 3. appearance, function 4. crooked 5. crowding 6. malocclusion 7. treatment plan 8. removable, fixed 9. headgear 10. retainer

Read 2

1. F 2. T 3. F 4. F 5. F 6. F

Read 3

1. *orthos* means straight or proper and *odous* means tooth 2. malocclusion 3. two types : removable and fixed 4. made of metal and sometimes of plastic or ceramic 5. a retainer

Listening

1. orthodontics 2. crooked 3. appliances 4. headgear 5. patient

Part 3 : Dialogue

Keywords

smile (2) crooked (5) crowding (16) taken out (4) extract (10) severity (8) adjusting (15) braces (9) removable (11) permanent (17) sugary food (12) dental hygienist (14) lifestyle (3) hard food (6) sticky food (13) plaque (1) retainers (7)

Question focus

1. Can I have orthodontic treatment 2. have any teeth taken out 3. will the treatment take 4. to visit the dental clinic 5. braces are available 6. for my teeth and braces 7. change my lifestyle 8. orthodontic treatment permanent

2) Listening

1. (2) 2. (4) 3. (5) 4. (1) 5. (7) 6. (6) 7. (3)

Word stew

orthodontics crooked crowding malocclusion braces

● 83

6. Dental Trauma

Part 1 : Vocabulary

1) trauma (6) cheeks (2) jawbones (8) fractured (12) extrusion (1) avulsed (15) swollen (10) painful (14) bloody (13) knocked out (7) socket (3) crown (11) root (5) saline (9) moist (4)

4) 1. trauma 2. fractured 3. knocked out 4. swollen 5. reimplanted

Read 1

1. accidents 2. contact 3. fractured 4. avulsed 5. swollen 6. cold compress 7. quickly 8. crown 9. root 10. moist

Read 2

1. F 2. T 3. T 4. F 5. T 6. F 7. F 8. F

Read 3

1. contact sports 2. an avulsed tooth 3. if they have deep cuts 4. it will die 5. in the patient's mouth

Listening

1. fractured 2. extrusion 3. concussion 4. intrusion 5. avulsed

Part 3 : Dialogue

Keywords

fracture (6) knock out (13) accident (8) sports injury (2) lips (12) swelling (14) bleeding (7) in a state of shock (3) pass out (11) lost consciousness (9) accident and emergency unit (16) reimplant (1) moist (4) saliva (15) scrub (10) rinse (5)

Question focus

1. How does that usually happen 2. patients have any other problems 3. feel immediately after the accident 4. should be done 5. what should you do 6. tooth that has been knocked out 7. keep a knocked-out tooth 8. if the tooth is dirty

2) Listening

1. (4) 2. (2) 3. (6) 4. (7) 5. (1) 6. (5) 7. (8) 8. (3)

Word stew

trauma fractured swollen knocked out reimplant

7. Tooth Whitening

Part 1 : Vocabulary

1) cosmetic dentistry (3) discoloration (7) enamel (5) stained (1) tetracycline (9) in-office bleaching (10) chairside bleaching (11) at-home bleaching (15) over-the-counter (8) mouth tray (14) bleaching gel (13) side effects (12) sensitivity (6) irritation (4) hydrogen peroxide (2)

4) 1. enamel 2. mouth tray 3. protective gel 4. prescribe 5. gingival irritation

Read 1
1. dissatisfied 2. cosmetic 3. Discoloration 4. stained 5. chairside 6. over-the-counter 7. tray 8. prescribe 9. sensitivity 10. irritation

Read 2
1. T 2. F 3. F 4. T 5. F 6. F 7. T 8. T 9. T 10. T

Read 3
1. 10,000 2. it becomes less porous 3. There are 3 options : in-office bleaching, at-home bleaching, OTC products 4. in-office bleaching 5. in the mouth tray 6. between 30 minutes and an hour 7. there are 2 side effects : mild-to-moderate tooth sensitivity and gingival irritation

Listening
1. 34 2. 100,000 3. 10, 5 4. 15, 30 5. 1, 3 6. 30, 2, 4 7. 60

Part 3 : Dialogue

Keywords
stained (2) treatment (6) mouth tray (11) prescribe (3) hydrogen peroxide (13) sensitivity (5) side effect (12) gums (8) teeth (1) sensitive (10) whiter (14) brush (4) dental floss (7) dental hygienist (15) maintenance (9)

Question focus
1. What are the differences between 2. treatment painful 3. any side effects 4. whiter will my teeth get 5. will my teeth stay white 6. How much does

2) Listening
1. (2) 2. (1) 3. (6) 4. (3) 5. (7) 6. (5) 7. (4)

Word stew
1. whitening 2. sensitivity 3. side effects 4. prescribe 5. stained

【著者略歴】

Jeremy Williams (ジェレミー・ウィリアムス)

トリニティ音楽大学大学院修了後, シェフィールド大学大学院で日本経済と現代文化を専門に研究. 現在, 東京医科大学国際医学情報学分野の主任教授を務めながら, 日本の研究と学識を世界に幅広く広めるため活動中.

After graduating Trinity College of Music, Jeremy Williams studied Japanese economics and modern Japanese culture at Sheffield University. Currently, he is the Professor and Chair of the Department of International Medical Communications at Tokyo Medical University, in which capacity he is dedicated to helping disseminate Japanese research and knowledge to a global audience.

C.S. Langham (クライブ・ラングハム)

英国出身. 1980年にケント大学大学院応用言語学科を修了.

インドネシアや中東などで教育に従事したのち, 1985年に来日. 日本では多くの国立・私立大学で教鞭を執り, 現在では日本大学歯学部教授 (外国語・英語). 研究分野は科学英語 (Scientific English) と発表言語 (the language of presentations). 全国語学教育学会 (JALT) と日本医学英語教育学会 (JASMEE) に所属.

Clive Langham is from the UK and is a graduate of the Applied Linguistics program at the University of Kent. He has worked in Indonesia and the Middle East. He came to Japan for the first time in 1985 and has worked at a number of national and private universities. He is currently a professor at Nihon University, school of dentistry. His field is Applied Linguistics. His major research interest is scientific discourse. He is a member of the Japan Association of Language Teachers and the Society for Medical English Education. He has published a number of books on presentations and dental English.

<ruby>井上<rt>いのうえ</rt></ruby> <ruby>孝<rt>たかし</rt></ruby>

1978 年	東京歯科大学卒業
1983 年	カナダトロント大学歯学部客員助教授（1985 年 8 月まで）
1994 年	アメリカアラバマ大学歯学部客員研究員（1994 年 4 月まで）
2001 年	東京歯科大学教授
2009 年	東京歯科大学口腔科学研究センター所長
2010 年	東京歯科大学大学院研究科長
2013 年	東京歯科大学千葉病院長
	東京歯科大学歯科衛生士専門学校校長
2019 年	東京歯科大学名誉教授・特任教授
2022 年	東京医学技術専門学校・校長
2024 年	姫路歯科衛生専門学校・校長

　大学卒業後，カナダトロント大学に長期留学し英会話の重要性を痛感し積極的に同世代の仲間と酒を飲み話をした．その後アラバマ大学に短期留学したがトロント時代に学んだ英語力は問題なく研究や生活の中で使うことができるようになっていた．大学では，国際渉外部長として姉妹校締結に，留学生の受け入れに貢献し，2007 年からは公用語を英語とする FDI（世界歯科機構）の理事として，職務をこなすことができた．現在 AI の進歩で翻訳機能を持つ PC も多くあるが，コミュニケーションに英語力は必須であると考える．

　臨床写真を提供して頂きました，矢島安朝先生，武田孝之先生，土肥福子先生，根津 崇先生に深謝いたします．

※本書は2011年11月に「English for the Dental Clinic 歯科医院で使える英語 音声CD付」として発行されたものを，内容は発行時のまま，音声データをCDではなく，小社WEBサイトを通じて提供する形式に変更したうえで，再発行したものです．

English for the Dental Clinic
歯科医院で使える英語
音声DL付　　　　　　　　　　　　　　　ISBN978-4-263-45689-7

2025年1月20日　第1版第1刷発行

著者代表　Jeremy Williams
発行者　白　石　泰　夫
発行所　医歯薬出版株式会社

〒113-8612　東京都文京区本駒込1-7-10
TEL.（03）5395-7638（編集）・7630（販売）
FAX.（03）5395-7639（編集）・7633（販売）
https://www.ishiyaku.co.jp/
郵便振替番号 00190-5-13816

乱丁，落丁の際はお取り替えいたします　　印刷・木元省美堂／製本・皆川製本所
Ⓒ Ishiyaku Publishers, Inc., 2025. Printed in Japan

本書の複製権・翻訳権・翻案権・上映権・譲渡権・貸与権・公衆送信権（送信可能化権を含む）・口述権は，医歯薬出版㈱が保有します．
本書を無断で複製する行為（コピー，スキャン，デジタルデータ化など）は，「私的使用のための複製」などの著作権法上の限られた例外を除き禁じられています．また私的使用に該当する場合であっても，請負業者等の第三者に依頼し上記の行為を行うことは違法となります．

JCOPY ＜出版者著作権管理機構 委託出版物＞
本書をコピーやスキャン等により複製される場合は，そのつど事前に出版者著作権管理機構（電話 03-5244-5088，FAX 03-5244-5089，e-mail：info@jcopy. or. jp）の許諾を得てください．